MEDIOCRE MOM MAGIC!

10 WAYS IMPERFECTION WILL BRING YOU MORE JOY AND EASE

TESSA ARANDA

Mediocre Mom Magic: 10 Ways Imperfection Will Bring You More Joy and Ease

Copyright © 2023 Tessa Aranda

Cover designed by Tessa Aranda

This book is a consolidation of my work as a Master Spark Coaching Facilitator for moms for over a decade. All great work is built on the shoulders of giants, and all ideas herein have been formulated from the works of various brilliant thinkers, coaches, and artist cited on page 130

Illustration Credits appear on page 132

Tessa Aranda
  Visit my website at
  www.MediocreMomsClub.com

Printed in the United States of America
First Printing: March 2023

Roots & Branches Publishing

ISBN-9798386026417

Dedication

To my girls. May you know that mastering your mediocrity is what makes you
the most magical human.

Contents

Mediocre motherhood is a new magical way of being. Owning your mediocrity allows space to create more in this world and contribute more value not less.

-Tessa Aranda

1. WHY MED

¡OCRITY?

Here's Why

BECAUSE IT'S LIBERATING TO y'all! Taking back the ickiest self-squashing doubts in our head that we're not the best so we might as well not try!? Yeah. Goodbye!

Guess what, mediocrity has no more negative connotations. It belongs to the beautifully messy, gorgeously ordinary, miraculously mundane moments of this thing we call life. And who are its champions? Who are the warriors that from the kitchen sinks of life rise up in majestical joy filled glory? Mothers. Society's unicorns of possibility with magical powers of creating something out of nothing, taking naps anytime, anywhere, and habit stacking like a boss (we're also taking back the word multitasking and all the negative connotations it's come to take on. Habit stacking y'all.)

Here is where your journey to freedom begins. Owning your mediocrity allows space to create more in this world and contribute more value not less. Mediocrity is a gift to yourself as a woman and a mother for experiencing grace in your life. Embracing mediocrity invites inspiration in place of shut down when faced with a desire. It allows that desire to expand your possibilities and your vision instead of feeding the 'I'm not good enough'. Mediocre motherhood is not a dig, it is a new magical way of being. Mastering mediocrity is the answer for mothers to have and do and be more in their lives.

Contemporary studies are finding that mothers who set realistic and achievable goals for themselves, rather than striving for perfection and success, are happier and less stressed (no shocker right? I'm just that little birdie in your head here with those reminders!). There are other studies that say moms who practice daily mindfulness and self-compassion have lower levels of depression and anxiety and are deliciously satisfied with their lives and their power to create the life they want. The key for these women? Focusing on the present moment and finding joy in the everyday activities of motherhood, rather than constantly striving for doing more.

And as a mother of 5 and a lifelong creative, do you know what I'm really great at, now? Being mediocre. I always was- but I was miserable because I refused to accept it. Did you ever feel like the almost best all-star on your team as a kid? The gracious and 'it's ok I didn't really care anyway' runner up in anything? The contributor to some creative endeavor with the most 'potential'? Barf right? I hated being told when I was young how much potential I had. Joy and fulfillment of my quest was only supposed to come if I was the best. The winner.

And I am fully aware that being a Master of Mediocrity seems like an oxy-moron. Until it doesn't. How can someone be exceptional at something that is clearly defined as low quality, low value, ordinary?

It has always been this way for me. I was a very precocious child. Intelligent. Teacher's pet. Things came easily to me, at least in the classroom, and oftentimes athletically. My brain moved too fast, was always creating, and always on to the next thing. So the inevitable results of not checking my work, getting bored of a task I had to repeat frequently, or overthinking something in front of me that was very face value was, I was never the best. There was always someone exceptional, committed, focused. And that was not me.

I was praised for being wildly creative (when that was allowed in the circumstance), uplifting, thinking outside the box. But in a society that values order and hierarchical achievement, that did not give me the top slot. And the problem was. I wanted the top. Maybe you wanted to disappear into the wallpaper when it came to academics, but I know for every woman there is that one place in their life where being just the 'less valuable' choice felt like crap.

I wanted to succeed on their terms. I was not *quite* creative and different enough to be that outlier. That entrepreneurial or inventive genius. That kid who totally flunked school but devoured books on their interests with a vice-like obsession while not giving a crap what people said and knowing I was going to do this thing. You know, like the Elon Musks, the Steve Jobs', the Oprah Winfreys of the world.

I remember vividly in first grade, after the 1994 Olympics, going ice-skating for the first time. It was blissful... I could do a turn, hold my foot up a beat. And I remember on the car ride home the devastation and frustration that my parents did not put me in ice skates at 18 months old and have me coached 5 days a week so that I would, obviously, be on my way to Olympic greatness. I was behind. Already. At 7 years old.

Years later, over my last decade as a marketer and marketing mindset coach, I spent years in the churn of the current 'achievement' current online. Do more. Hustle harder. Hold to your vision. If it's not being created you are not doing hard enough things. Believing enough. Holding your vision enough. You are never going to be enough. And that's what drives you. I always could feel it but one day I woke up and owned it. I don't want to be them. Ever. And that's ok. And suddenly the recognition of that truth set me free. Are you ready to stop comparing, stop feeling as if you've fallen short and find your mediocre genius? Let's go discover your Joy.

MEDIOCRE (lame, modern defn.)

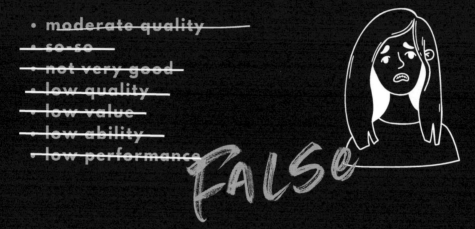

- ~~moderate quality~~
- ~~so-so~~
- ~~not very good~~
- ~~low quality~~
- ~~low value~~
- ~~low ability~~
- ~~low performance~~

False

MEDIOCRE (revolutionary motherhood defn.)

beautifully messy, gorgeously
ordinary, miraculously mundane

True

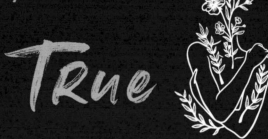

DISCOVERING MY JOY

It is difficult to find happiness within oneself, but it is impossible to find it anywhere else

- Arthur Schopenhauer

STRIVING FOR IMPERFECTION SAVED me. If you've ever experienced crippling anxiety, you might get when I say that I was dying inside, and what brought me back to life? Intentionally attempting imperfect action, daily.

Just 9 years ago, during my third pregnancy, I was so riddled with stress and impulsive, fight-or-flight action that it all came to a head. Through my constant go go go, I began to fight a fatigue unlike anything I had ever experienced before. In the midst of doing some huge project I undertook and had piled pressure on myself to complete, I had my first full blown panic attack. And then they came more frequently. Anxiety was not something that happened to me, it was a full on way of being. I remember the room spinning regularly and wondering if this happens to other mothers. If they have to take deep breaths for the world to just hold still long enough to get your bearings and get up again.

My entire life I have been driven. I have wanted to create, to do, to be more. I am talented. But never the best. 'You have so much potential, 'You are so creative you are going to do amazing things', 'You are so strong from what you've been through' and then, from my college therapist, 'Because of your tendencies [to be a spaz and incapacity to emotionally regulate, is what she meant], you shouldn't ever have more than one or two kids'. Way to throw a wrench in my plans for creative world domination lady. (not to mention the 4 kids I had always dreamed of).

Eventually, I was diagnosed with adrenal fatigue, suffered through 6 years of postpartum and prenatal depression before being diagnosed and receiving help, and at the end of this particular pregnancy, a wildly miserable case of shingles. [which in case you didn't know, is triggered by stress]. I had to stop. I had to find a new way of operating. There was no instant pill, but magic began to slowly seep into my life and my way of being through slight shifts in my perception. Through not just accepting my Mediocrity- but embracing and loving it, and then getting comfortable taking wildly imperfect steps forward.

Throughout the next 6 years, intentionally slowing down and learning the skills and tools that I am going to share with you here completely changed me as a person. This is not some just, like, fun little saying at the beginning of a book. 6 years ago, I was rage-filled, overwhelmed, and resentful with a deep, pervasive sense of hopelessness in motherhood.

I am not perfect. But I am better because I have learned surrender and imperfect action. I feel better. I have come to embody the tools I have learned, like how to quickly shift when I screw up, and how to bring back the magic for me and anyone involved. I'm sure you have experienced this, that crippling hamster wheel of self-talk and self-doubt, wondering why you screwed that circumstance up so badly and how you could have done it differently. But guess what? When you learn these keys of radical self-awareness, the mistakes make the magic. That's truly how accepting and loving your mediocrity can come to affect your life, and this profound perspective realignment is my deepest desire for you.

The following chapters are written to be morsels of soul food for the ordinary mother. They have been arranged in such a way that they may be read in one sitting in just a few hours one after the other, building on each other and giving you deeper and greater awareness into your character and potential as a master mediocre mother. And they also have been written so that you can send pen at any time to any page, and receive a bite of hope, or a nibble of enthusiasm, igniting pings of inspiration for new ways of being in your own motherhood and life. [and it's small enough to fit into your purse! Wink wink]

My intention with this book is not to give you some formula and a new list of things to-do.

My intention is to invite you to receive a shift in perspective around your sub-par humanity. Your slip-ups, your almost made-it's, your continual I-should-have-done-better. To take back the power from your flaws and embrace them as your strengths. And begin to see the divine in the ordinary of your life. The magic in the divinely mediocre of your days, your achievements, your efforts... and unlock the power in your mothering in a way that has the potential to magnify all of the good that every single human in your home has to offer.

Come with me.

THE MEDIOCRE MOTHER'S JOURNEY

This book takes you through the process of embracing and magnifying your mediocraty for the purpose of creating a life you crave. It's important to note that this process has no care for if you currently love how ordinary you feel or you absolutely hate the perceived mundane of your life. In both cases, the path with offer you something of value

NEW WAY OF THINKING

1. WHY MEDIOCRITY?
2. EXTRA-ORDINARY
3. RESTORATION VS. REST

Mmm…Appetizers to disrupt moms' "glorification of busy" status quo. Take some tasty bites to become a believer baby! When you believe (in the magic of mediocrity) you receive. And there's so much goodness in ending the battle of "enoughness" in your brain once and for all.

NEW WAY OF BEING

4. MOM WHO YOU ARE
5. DO VS. BE
6. VISIONARY

Imbibe in these Tasty Morsels to feel your inner voice shift as you expand your self-awareness & capacity for joy. As you work through this section with me, you'll toss out those expired, negative beliefs. Who needs em?! Not. Us. Because it's the golden age of authentic motherhood and moms have the power to have more, be more, create more, while doing less. Mkay?! Repeat after me: "I have the capacity to create what I desire with joy & ease." Ahhh. Tranquility baby.

NEW WAY OF DOING

7. FUNCOMFORTABLE
8. BIG FUN
9. PROCESS OVER PERFECTION
10. FIND THE MAGIC

Dessert. Mmmm yesss finally dessert. Dripping, gooey, thick deliciousness that makes the mouth water… ok I'll stop. This is where we unleash the magic. Where you begin to "do" from a place of custard-ed up "believe-in-myself-so-hard" gooey goodness. The perfect ending to a delicious filling meal for your serenity starved soul.

2.YOU DONT BE EXTRAO

HAVE TO

RDINARY

Become "Extra" At Being Ordinary

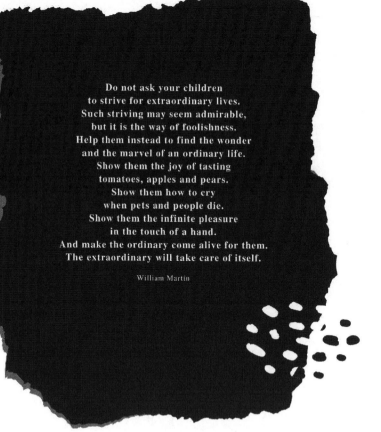

Do not ask your children
to strive for extraordinary lives.
Such striving may seem admirable,
but it is the way of foolishness.
Help them instead to find the wonder
and the marvel of an ordinary life.
Show them the joy of tasting
tomatoes, apples and pears.
Show them how to cry
when pets and people die.
Show them the infinite pleasure
in the touch of a hand.
And make the ordinary come alive for them.
The extraordinary will take care of itself.

William Martin

WHAT IF EXTRAORDINARY WAS not something that we strive for anymore, but instead became something that we discovered? Something that IN the ordinary, 'took care of itself.' Now, don't get me wrong I do not believe in stagnancy, staying still, complacency. So don't get it twisted. I just believe that there isn't as much force necessary for progress than most of us have been conditioned to believe. The fun part is, finding the magic in the mediocre is all about being 'extra'.

The extraordinary often requires one path. One way. Unyielding focus. Athletes are a prime example, becoming the best in their sport after daily intensive repetition and training. Following the one single path to greatness. But the fabulous thing about being ordinary is there are a million paths to being extra at it. The opportunity to be extra at being ordinary is available to us at nearly every moment, in any circumstance, in any state. Want to be the most 'extra' ordinary mom on a rainy day? See the magic in the moment and encourage the quest for the most epic puddle jump. Want to be the most 'extra' ordinary friend? Belt her a birthday song in all your pitchy glory at that girls night out. Want to be the most 'extra' wife on date night? Google those Cosmo kissing tricks and laugh your way through the silliest, most novel makeout sesh you've had in years. You getting the idea?

My best friend Arielle once said to me, *"Your mediocre singing is my favorite. Because it makes me feel like I can do anything- for no reason. That I can choose to do things just because those things make me happy. And I've been holding myself back from doing things I love because I am not great."*

So how do we become more 'extra'. How do we make it natural to embrace and magnify our ordinary so that the inevitable magic and joy will unfold? The first step is to begin to believe it is in the ordinary that all of the greatest magic in this world lives. Then, to see it more often. We can not magnify when we don't even know where to look or what we are looking at.

Have you ever been wildly inspired by cheering for the underdog? The unextraordinary? The person that wasn't the best? That didn't win? Why? We live in a society that values achievement and mastery and rarely gives much recognition to the ordinary. Do you ever remember a time when the celebration of the ordinary was more profound and powerful in moving you to feelings and action than the expectation of achievement? Sports movies do this well, actually.

Have you heard the story of the One Love Bowl? In 2008, a high school football game took place between Gainesville State School and Grapevine Faith in Texas? The head coach of Grapevine Faith, Kris Hogan, decided to do something special for the opposing Gainesville team. He asked half of his fans to cheer for the Tornadoes and even had half of the cheerleaders root for them. The game was played, and the Gainesville players heard their names shouted from the stands for possibly the first time in their lives. They were confused that the families and community were asking them to hit their kids, and for them to score and possibly win over their own team.

Why did this happen, and why were the players so confused? Well, because Gainesville was a maximum-security correctional facility, and the players were all teenagers with convictions for crimes such as drugs, assault, and robbery. Grapevine Faith, on the other hand, was a well-established football team with 11 coaches and the latest equipment. The enthusiastic energy was palpable as the Gainesville boys were buoyed up by the belief of their own cheering fans. Belief in their efforts and their worthiness that possibly no one had ever shown them before.

In the end, though they didn't win, they scored two touchdowns, playing the best game of their lives. After the game, both teams gathered in the middle of the field to pray, and one of the Gainesville players led the prayer, thanking God saying that he never would have known that a single person cared if it weren't for this experience at this game.

On their way back to the bus, each player was given a bag with food, a Bible, and an encouraging letter from a Grapevine Faith player. The game has had a lasting impact on Gainesville, with the leaders of the facility saying the spirit at the juvenile detention facility has completely changed.

The reason this story brings us to tears is not because we're the hugest football fans (or maybe you are), but because a piece of our soul recognizes that in celebration, recognition, and love of the not-so-extraordinary—- we begin to see what actually is. That in every ordinary moment- there is the possibility of magic.

What is extraordinary? What is extraordinary is the determination of those Gainesville boys to continually show up for their team, game after game, even though they always lost. What's extraordinary were the ordinary actions of the few hundred Grapevine fans who made a profound difference in the lives of many.

You do not have to be extraordinary. I give you permission right now to claim—- with bright celebration—- your profound ordinary-ness. 'I am NOT EXTRAORDINARY!' Shout it! Outloud. Right now. I'm serious. (No but for real you'll learn more about this in part 7- ha!) I proclaim and shout from the rooftops, that moving forward with an eye toward growth, toward expansion, and becoming more of who you want to be, in a way that is purposely imperfect- you will shine brighter in your ordinariness than you ever have by feeling down about how not extraordinary you are.

In my own life this declaration has allowed me to expand my influence and impact. For years I was singing live on social media and inspiring through my often off-key efforts. I was consistently thanked for showing up in my pitchy glory. For being uninhibited and in love with the moment.I was naturally creating and living in a magic that I couldn't understand how to teach until I began to fully embrace and obsess over the ordinary.

The irony is that the obsession that I found for living an ordinary life is what helped me finally achieve the get-the-stu-pid-thing-you-love-done-even-if-it's-messy I have been striving for for over a decade. (My dream of Publishing a book for moms and launching my podcast—it's all here! And I got to create it with such Ease!) Do those obscure things that spark life in you. Relent to the compulsion to create. Embrace obsessions. Fall deep down the rabbit hole of your fascination. Trust your curiosity to birth whatever is sparking an uprising in your soul. And then, if we're not going to live striving for perfection anymore, for the unreachable extraordinary, then what do we do now?

Read on my friend. Let's dig into some tools for unlocking your 'extra'.

THE PATH TO EXTRAORDINARY

BEING "EXTRA" AT BEING ORDINARY

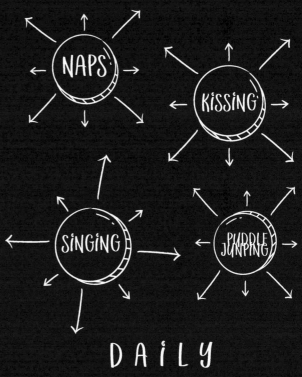

LIFETIME

NAPS

KISSING

SINGING

PUDDLE JUMPING

DAILY

(MOMENT TO MOMENT)

3. RESTORA

TION VS. REST

THE LIFE GIVING CYCLE

WHAT IF YOU COULD start your day truly, deeply rested? Ready to take on the world with a deep sense of pulsating life force? What the heck is that? I don't know. It's like jumping up in the morning without the alarm with a pep in your step as you sprint to the toilet for your morning pee. Maybe even whilst whistling a happy little tune on the pot instead of...uh. Falling asleep there again? What? You thought that was just you? Toilet sleeping? Nah.

What if you were not just **not** tired... you were inspired, daily. Oooooh yeah! What would you do to have this? Instead of constantly chasing 'more rest' (Will there ever be enough?), we can attain that delicious feeling of renewal by creating a practice of restoration. Every time I shift into this, everything in my world changes. And honestly, I have to get knocked down and reminded again and again to get back on this restoration practice bandwagon. It's easy to start, fun to maintain, but y'all - life happens and I don't know anyone who keeps the flippin habit up forever. But that doesn't matter. Once you learn this, practice it, and feel the results, you'll be able to recalibrate and use it over and over for the rest of todos dias. That means forever, y'all.

Here's the life changing truth: Rest Comes in the Morning! Let me explain. Tell me, does this happen to you? You're so mentally exhausted from your day, from putting out fires, chasing the next most urgent thing, attempting moments of 'me', exercising, friends, that podcast you love... not to mention the constant interruptions and explosions of chaos...

Then when bedtime comes you are so ready to rest. As you collapse into your bed, you attempt to shut out the world, your responsibilities, the 'more' you constantly need to do, with something that can drown your thoughts.

You attempt to just sleep - but it comes in fits as your husband lays there peacefully snoring his head off, while you're stuck battling blips of anxiety that keep you from drifting off for what seems like hours...

TV, social media, YouTube... whatever fits the bill for the night for you to release and not be needed... to not have to think and decide or respond for just one minute... only that minute turns into hours. You cannot even believe what time it is... only now you're not tired. Maybe sometimes you find a strategy that works. Sex, a good book - you may even find some powerful audio visualizations. But it never lasts. Eventually, it comes back. That unrelenting exhaustion. Because that time alone - to be the only one demanding of your attention - is precious.

So how can you have both? Self-focused restoration while still getting sleep that you need to survive and function? Cuz y'all, I tried that 5am power hour crap and I quit. I believe in chronotypes (google it) and we are not all made to be most high-functioning (or functioning at all) at the butt crack of when the sun's not even out yet.

So here's the deal: If you want to not only feel rested but ignited each day of your life, this is the truth. True, deep, replenishing rest comes in the morning, because without a daily restoration, we never absorb that rest we so desperately need and crave. I hear my mom-friends screaming at me through the book already. But this is God's honest truth. You simply cannot fall into rest at the end of the day, if sometime at the beginning of it, you did not have time to be still, to be alone (at least in your thoughts), and to restore.

Girl - this does not have to be complicated. And it doesn't need to be all or nothing either. Dog needs to walk? Habit stack. Strap him in, get your steps, feel the sunshine on your skin, and partake of some spiritual soul food (in the form of books, worship, music, podcasts, etc.). Telling me your kids wake up and breathe down your neck from the crack of dawn? Noise canceling headphones were my best investment ever. Do you know what one of my favorite restorative morning practices is? Kitchen dancing. Cleaning up totally 'alone'. They might be talkin' but I ain't hearin'! I inform my children to only disturb me in case of a dire emergency and get their morning stuff done in a timely manner while I work. Alone while together.

The yummiest form of morning restoration, of course, comes when you can practice stillness, breathwork, guided meditations, maybe even some in-depth journaling. But y'all, if you can't get it done before the kids get up and the day is in full swing,make it happen later anyway. Don't throw out the baby with the bath water! Schedule. IT. IN. Force yourself to stick with it. My rule of thumb is if I can schedule and get it done before noon, I completed my restoration by the end of the morning. And then - ohhhhh what magic unfolds!

Restoration and rest are cyclical. They will always feed one another. As you practice restoration, your rest will change. You will approach bedtime differently, experiencing a greater sense of fulfillment or completion in your day, and an ease as you slip away to sleep. As your rest becomes more re-energizing, you have more to give to your morning practice of daily restoration, and on, and on, and on, until you're the crazy one telling every mom who will listen that 'You don't need more rest! You need restoration in the morning!'

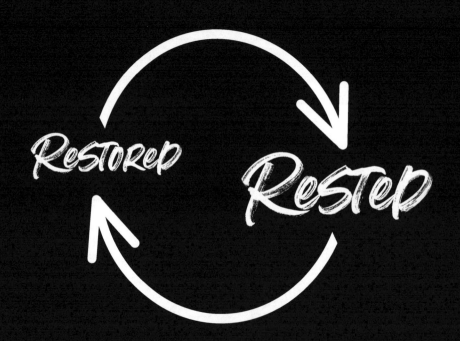

The Magic Void

THE MAGIC VOID IS a time of rest, reflection, and recharge that can lead to creative growth and manifestation. The idea is that in order to tap into our full potential and bring our creative ideas to life, we need to make space for stillness, introspection, and rejuvenation. The void is what actually begets creation. I mean, how unproductive and in survival mode do you feel when you are pregnant? Such a grand example for this time of stillness, rest, receiving before the birth of new life.

Another incredible metaphor for this time is the 'fallow' period when a field is left without crops to be grown. In a field that is drained, depleted, and starved of nutrients, this period allows for recovery of the soil's fertility, the reduction of the buildup of pests and diseases, and the conservation of moisture. By taking a break from planting crops, farmers are able to prepare the soil for future crop production and improve the overall health of their fields. All of nature exsists in these cycles; seasons, menses, lunar cycles, migrations. Why do we not allow the break in expectations and demands to be emptied and improve the health of our hearts?

This 'magic void' allows us to connect with our inner wisdom, gain clarity on our desires and goals, and align our actions with what truly matters to us. In other words, taking a break from our daily routines, and a break from our 'big fun' goals (see Part 8) when inspiration runs dry, giving ourselves permission to pause, can help us reap the benefits of a refreshed and refocused mind.

Creation happens as a result of natural cycles and the need for rest, renewal, and reflection. For mediocre mamas looking for a more vibrant life, these periods of emptiness and stillness can help mothers tap into their creativity, gain new insights and perspectives, and replenish their energy levels. By embracing these moments of stillness, mothers can re-emerge with fresh ideas, a clearer focus, and a greater sense of joy and fulfillment. Essentially, the magic void period is a time to slow down, reconnect with yourself, and allow the creative mind to flourish.

Often, when feeling creatively stumped or energetically drained, we pile on guilt or even shame around what we should be doing - if we pause, we will continue to lose motivation, forward growth, and we will never be able to get out of it. We dread the uninspired spiral..

'Will I always feel this way?'

I'm sure you've experienced this lack of zest for life at some point in your motherhood, and likely felt like something must be wrong, and you must fight it. But what if everything was exactly as it should be?

The biggest disservice to women is not educating us on cycles, on the true nature of our being, and the rhythms that we follow just like the Earth - that the fallow is the magic. It is divine. And all we must do is surrender to it. We must rewrite what we are allowed to feel in a pause. Not that we must get up. Not that we are failing. Not that we will be swallowed up in it. And that at different seasons and with different focuses of our lives, the void may be short or long, huge or so small we might not even notice it.

What is possible to feel in this magic void? Excited anticipation through releasing pressure to do or to produce and relaxing with gratitude for the expectation of emergence. The pause still requires you to continue feeding your soul. It is a time of feast, not famine. Just as the soil feasts on moisture and good bacteria in its necessary fallow, so can you feast on all of the mental, emotional, and spiritual nutrients in the pause. This is the magic of the void.

Shifting your heart from believing your void is a famine of your ability to give to beginning to see that you are feasting and becoming rich will change everything for you. We can relax into this period instead of trying to fight it. Like snuggling up next to a fire with a cozy blanket, a warm bowl of soup, and a good book in a snowstorm vs. shoveling your way through five feet of packed snow to get out to your favorite restaurant. The magic will always be in surrendering to the moment, the season, the rhythm. That is where all life begins.

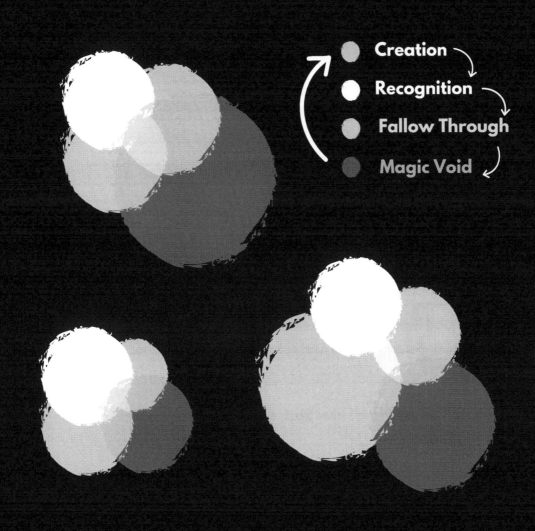

Creation

Recognition

Fallow Through

Magic Void

4. MOM WHO

YOU ARE

Values Over Strategies

ARE YOU READY TO tap into your inner greatness and discover your true north? It all starts with embracing who you already are. That's right, you don't need to reinvent the wheel, because you've already got a well-worn path that's uniquely yours. It's woven into every aspect of your life - from your interactions to your desires, successes, relationships, and even heartaches.

But hold on, before you hit the road to your next adventure, you need to know where you're starting from. It's like taking a road trip without knowing your current location - no GPS, no service, nada. How can you get to your destination if you don't know where you are? That's why it's crucial to discover your core values - that thread of 'who you are' that's been present throughout your entire life.

Now, take a look at the list above and highlight or circle any values that resonate with you. These are the things that are important to you, and that you've embodied all along. Then, through a process of elimination, narrow down your choices to the three most important or innate to who you are. Don't be tempted to choose things that sound good or that you wish you had. Your core values are the things that you already are and can experience often.

And here's the secret: once you know your core values, they become the rudder for steering the ship to more joy, more success, and more of what you want. You don't need to change who you are - you just need to embrace it fully and let your true self shine. So let's get started on this journey of discovering your magic and mastering your mediocrity. Share your chosen values in our group 'Mediocre Moms Club' (www.mediocremomsclub.com) and let's support each other on this incredible adventure!

ADVENTURE	GIVING	THOUGHTFULNESS	AFFECTION	FAITHFULNESS
FULFILLMENT	SUPPORT	COMMUNICATION	GRATITUDE	DEVOTION
BOLDNESS	SERVICE	UNDERSTANDING	PLEASURE	ENLIGHTENMENT
AMUSEMENT	IMPROVEMENT	WISDOM	WARMTH	ACCEPTANCE
COURAGE	CREATIVITY	LEADERSHIP	CONNECTION	RECEIVING
CONFIDENCE	VISION	CANDOR	FAMILY	APPRECIATION
ENJOYMENT	IMAGINATION	DIRECTION	COMMUNITY	ACKNOWLEDGMENT
BEAUTY	RESOURCEFULNESS	MASTERY	COOPERATION	CARING
GRACE	ORIGINALITY	AUTHENTICITY	ALIGNMENT	WELCOMING
RADIANCE	EXPANSION	INFLUENCE	INTIMACY	ACCOMPLISHMENT
ELEGANCE	INNOVATION	ENCOURAGEMENT	LOVE	ACHIEVEMENT
EXCELLENCE	DISCOVERY	SINCERITY	FUN	COMPLETION
MAGNIFICENCE	LEARNING	CLARITY	COMPASSION	REALIZATION
INSPIRATION	CONTEMPLATION	TOUCH	PRESENCE	SUCCESS
MOTIVATION	INSIGHT	EXCELLENCE	DELIGHT	EFFICIENCY
INTUITION	REFINEMENT	UNDERSTANDING	FREEDOM	HARMONY
AWARENESS	DISCERNMENT	EFFECTIVENESS	CONNECTION	EASE
INSIGHT	REFLECTION	PROFICIENCY	ALIGNMENT	ORDER
OPENNESS	KNOWLEDGE	INTIMACY	CONSIDERATION	PEACEFULNESS
ENCOURAGEMENT	CLEVERNESS	COMMUNICATION	SPIRITUALITY	PREDICTABILITY
CONTRIBUTION	HONESTY	AUTHENTICITY	AWARENESS	TRANQUILITY
INTEGRITY	TRUTHFULNESS	PLAY	CONSCIOUSNESS	STABILITY

Here's an example, and a step by step for finding your own.

My CORE Three (Example):
When I first started using values to guide me I tried to choose my 3 core values. I circled things like adventure, confidence, amusement, grace, support, creativity, influence, inspiration, wisdom, clarity, tranquility, order, freedom, and discovery.

The State of Your Current Existence:
At this time I was living in circumstances that made me feel trapped, like I had no choice, I couldn't see a way out. I felt alone and overwhelmed often (my husband traveled for work and I had 4 kids under 6), and I was stumbling my way through motherhood and life. I was hopeful, I loved nature and could see the beauty in small moments. But the macro of my life felt like it was tumbling out of my control.

Who I Was Not:
With that state of my life in mind can you see how values I wanted like support, freedom, grace, order, and tranquility were aspirational values? Things that felt good to me because I wish I could experience them more often in the current state of my life? If I looked back at the thread of my existence from childhood, was I experiencing and allowing others to experience support everywhere I went? Not really. Clarity? No. Order? Definitely not.

Who I Was, Am, and Always Have Been:
But amusement. Oh yes. I was often amused by myself and could definitely knock some socks off of a crowd. This one is so normal to my way of existing it almost sounded boring. I don't want that, because I already have access to it anytime I want. Ohhhhhh. I already have it. I AM it. Bam. Found the thread. What about creativity? Heck, I don't remember a time in my life where I wasn't creating something and initiating the creation of others in some form or another. Boom. Me. Confidence? Heck yes. I was the chubby little 10 year old doing crazy dance moves for the diving contest at the public pool. No shame. Total freedom and self-love in whatever shape or form I found my body in my entire life, not to mention speaking up any and every time I felt inclined. Confidence was my jam. Is my jam.

Whittling it Down to Three:

Now, some of the other values are important to me *and* I can see throughout that thread of my life. Discovery, adventure, influence, inspiration, wisdom. And I may even cling to one or the other at different times when they feel more important. So, a powerful next step to whittle down to your three (and three is so important because our brain needs a finite focus when steering our path to what's next) is to ask others (from your list of the circled values) which ones are most innately you. Which ones do they experience when they are around you? Which values do they see as just being so core to who you are that they begin to feel more possibilities in their own life around that thing by being your friend? What are they inspired by when they see it in you?

Where Do You Want To Go?:

After receiving some of this optional feedback you can now ask yourself, what am I steering toward? Maybe at this time in your life you want your kids to feel better about themselves and become strong contributing members of the family and community. Maybe you want to create something you've been dreaming about for years or even decades. Maybe you want to find a way to start some powerful project for youth or working side by side with your kid or spouse to impact youth together. Maybe you want to feel more vibrant and focusing on completely transforming your health is your current focus. Whatever is 'next' for you can help you become clear on which of the things that you 'are' will keep you on the well worn path to where you are currently trying to go.

Example:

In my current mission to help mothers flip their 'not-enoughness' on its head and proudly harness their mediocrity to experience more joy and ease in their lives, I am able to utilize my 'beingness' of Amusement, Creativity, and Confidence to steer the ship to the impact I want to have in the world. Not only am I 'being' amusing, creative and confident in order to write and distribute this book, but in reading it, my readers are able to experience more joy, they find themselves being amused more easily, they see creative possibilities they hadn't been able to see before, and they begin to experience more confidence in who they are and have been their entire flippin lives. When I bring my core values into this space, it creates expansion for everyone. Hot dang! Isn't this so cool! This is real practical magic.

Momming Who You Are is key here because when you mom from a place of who you *should be* (forcing actions that feel contrary to who you are or what you are normally capable of) or from a place of *how you are* (the ebb and flow of feelings and emotions) the results are very different than anchoring ourselves into who we truly are at our core, and knowing that those are these exact gifts and ways of being that have prepared us to magnify the magical moments, problem solve in the difficult decisions l, and overcome our most frustrating mistakes.

THE TWO GENIUSES

THERE ARE TWO GENIUSES at work in your life. First, you are Genius. Second, you have a genius.

You Are a Genius

The first genius, the one that you Are, is what you are genius at being (everywhere, and it is not based on strategies, it is in everything you do). Your core values are the ones working their magic in your genius. Having a succinct, explicitly defined 'genius' is powerful in anchoring our identity and seeing what is possible. There is a specific process for finding your genius that I will not be outlining here in this book, because it is a powerful collaborative process that is available on . But understanding what it is and how you can utilize it is so important.

This genius can be utilized at any moment in any role, task or project. It is the essence of who you are and has been the consistent line of being throughout your life. Often, if we feel off while attempting some task, it is because we are attempting to be something we aspire to, or think we should be, instead of leveraging our innate genius, who we are. Your genius is usually a state of being that seems so mundane, so mediocre, so innate that others commend you for it but you generally count it for nothing. They think you are great but it's so easy for you and you are not the *best* at it so they're silly for commending you for it. Because it doesn't take much effort.

Have you ever heard the phrase: 'Teach us to be as amazing as you at [fill in the blank]...' and just laughed to yourself thinking... oh if this chick could only see how insanely imperfect I am, how impatient and rash, how unfocused and messy. This thing isn't that big of a deal, and I'm certainly not exceptional.' For me, this thing is creativity. It comes easily to me. It's also been hard to teach because the process for 'being' it since it is so natural to me. Once I went through the genius collaboration and discovered that my genius is *Cultivating Creation*, I realized that I don't need to figure out how to 'teach' creativity at all, or even be the best, most creative person in any one field. That I intrinsically cultivate the creativity in others and in the world around me by just being me! How freeing is that! You can just 'be' you and create more of the things that you want in this world! What if there was nothing to figure out? Nothing more you need to become. You already have and are everything you need. Ahhhhhhhh. Just sit in that a moment.

Magic right?

This is the power of the genius that was step one to completely transforming my striving. People who have gone through the genius collaboration find their genius is one of their core values with an action preceding it. *Facilitating Connection. Investigating Truth. Honoring Family. Unlocking Intimacy.*—- these are some of the 'geniuses' that have come out of the 'Genius Collaboration'. The power comes when the genius resonates so poignantly and powerfully with you that you could never forget it. That you feel buoyed up in seeing yourself in your strength in a way you never have before. In your greatness. Many express experiencing a swelling up into their chest upon the moment of discovering their genius that fills them to the brim and feels like bursting. Like they know themselves for the first time in their lives. Mmmmm. It's my favorite.

YOU'RE A "GENIUS" IN EVERYTHING

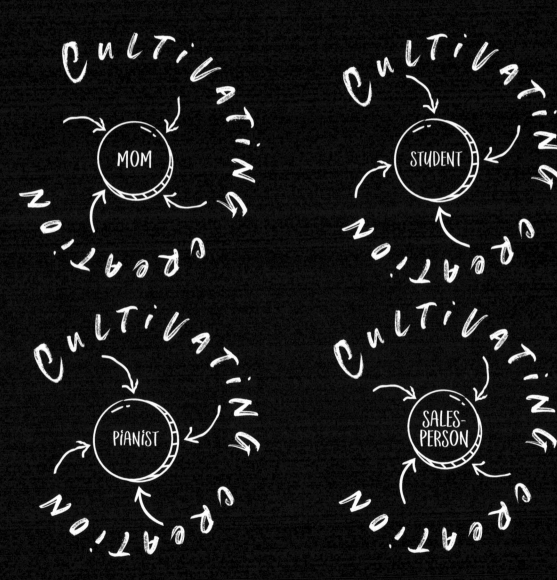

You Have a Genius

What is this second genius then? It's not the genius that you are, but the genius that you have! Crazy, right? Back in ancient Rome, they believed in this little sprite creature that would drop in and bestow inspiration, creativity, and flow. And get this, the word 'genius' comes from Latin meaning 'begetter' or 'attendant spirit'.

Nowadays, we tend to think of genius as something that people are, like if you make something cool or change your life in a big way, you must be some kind of superhuman. But that way of thinking does us a major disservice, my friend. Personally, I like to think of my genius as a rad little creature who's always on the lookout for ways to bring me some sweet goodness. A fun, bright, lovely little creature who's busy stocking up on brilliance to bring into my mind and heart when I am ready. I believe in the power of angels and spiritual guides as well as a Holy Spirit directed by God to inspire and reveal to me if and when I am ready to receive. Whatever form this creature (or multiple creatures) takes for you here lies the gift:

The important thing is that when we see our successes as gifts from a creative source outside of ourselves, we can be content no matter what. If we create something that sucks and gets a big ol' 'meh', we can just be like, 'oh well, my genius wasn't around today'. And if we create something amazing and get recognized for it, we can still say 'my genius was with me' and not get all high and mighty about it.

It's so freeing to be able to create without the pressure of judgment or the weight of success or failure. We can just focus on the process and take imperfect action every day. Plus, when we're open to receiving from a source outside of ourselves, we can experience more flow, joy, and ease in our lives.

Have you ever felt like you were hit with some otherworldly inspiration that couldn't possibly have come from you? How satisfying was the outcome? And if you haven't experienced it, think about how letting go of the responsibility for success or failure could help you create more.

There is no right or wrong answer, but as you continue to read through these magical morsels, I invite you to do so with the openness that you may in fact be visited by your genius. Take note of the magic that comes and the ease with which it was delivered to you.

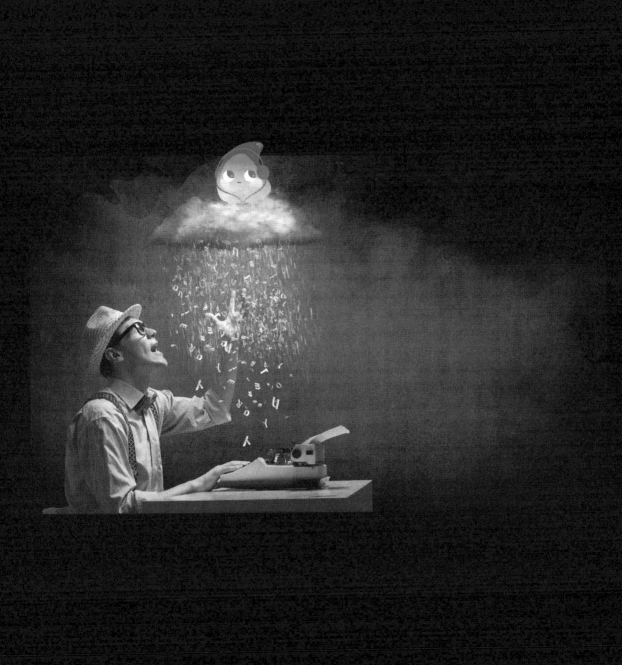

Receive Them & Lean In

HAVE YOU EVER FELT completely exhausted from meeting the demands of your family? The constant demands on your time, energy, and even your body can be overwhelming, right? What if instead of pushing away from your loved ones, you could stay true to your own schedule, desires, and goals while still being there for them? Being a mother is not an easy task, and it is normal to feel frustrated and overwhelmed with the never-ending responsibilities of motherhood.

As mothers, we often feel like targets of our children's constant needs and emotions, leaving us with little to no time to focus on ourselves. However, what if I told you that it is possible to shift from being a giver to a receiver for your children? To do this, we must first understand the value of receiving. For many of us, receiving love, compliments, and gifts can be challenging, and we may feel vulnerable and uncomfortable.

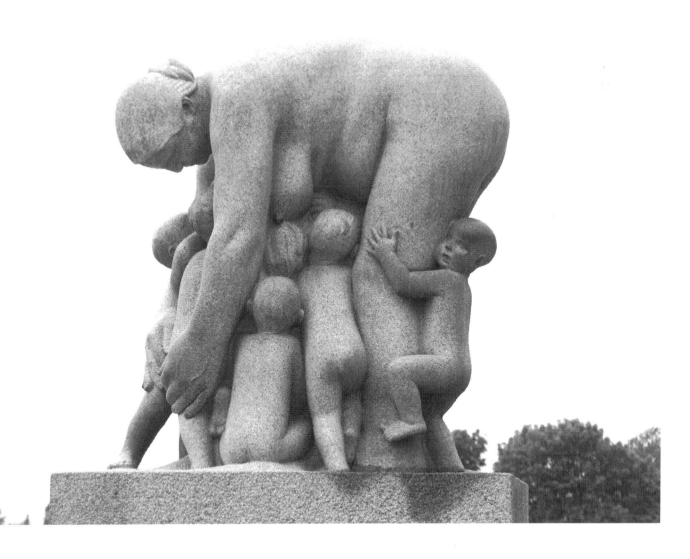

If you are good at receiving, it's likely that you had a nurturing parent who was great at receiving you. They created a safe space where you could just be yourself, without any fear of judgment. Unfortunately, not all of us had this kind of upbringing. Learning to receive can be challenging, but it is a practice that can make your life as a mother easier.

As mothers, we must learn to be aware of the distinction between giving and receiving. Being a safe harbor, a safe space where our children can empty themselves without us having to do anything about their emotions, is a divine role. You do not have to solve their problems or give in to their every whim. Your role is to be open, expansive, safe, and cozy for your children to rest their weary souls.

Once you are conscious of the distinction between receiving your children vs giving to your children, your ability to be aware in the moment and shift into an easy flow with each child's needs will completely change how drained you feel by the daily demands on you to give. This I can promise you.

Being a vessel is divinely designed. Being a safe harbor, a safe space to not have to *do* anything about our kids big emotions (and I'm talking feelings both enjoyable and in enjoyable here), to not have their emotions *mean* anything about us, to be open and available for our babies to empty themselves— and teach them to empty themselves to a higher power— is a divine role.

Some children seek to be heard and understood, while others may seek pity or physical interaction. The goal is not to quickly give in and attempt to 'fill them up' reactively, which only leaves them wanting more. Instead, we should aim to be intentional in our giving. Instead of giving them what they want, give them what they need. Lean in to what they need and they often need it for far less time than we believe, and it takes far less of our energy. When I forget to be in the intention of receiving with my family, I often remind myself that 'What I resist persists' and visualize myself as a receptacle.

Remember that wherever you are in your motherhood journey, you can be emptied and open to receive your children. You don't have to do more; all you need to do is understand this principle, and it will become easier for you to receive. Trust me; once you learn to receive, you'll begin to see miracles in your life as a mother.

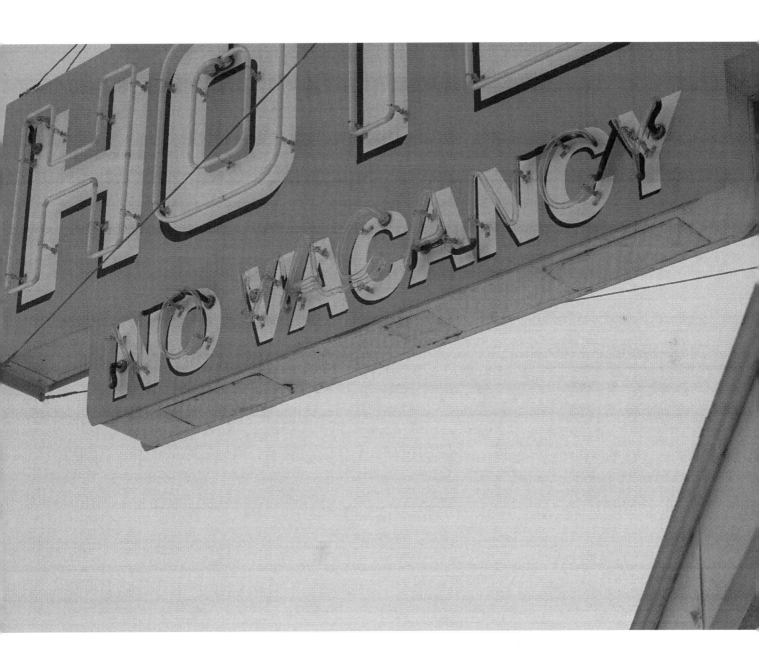

5. DO

VS. BE

Doing Motherhood or Being Mom

THERE'S A MISCONCEPTION THAT doing requires choice and that being is a consequence of that choice that happens to us. When I refer to 'being' I mean our disposition, our state of perceiving, understanding, and receiving the world around us. 'Being' is how we are in any given circumstance. How we feel, what we value, and how we perceive and respond to the world around us.

For example:

What I am doing (actions, behaviors): riding a ferris wheel. How I am being (feel, experiencing): giddy, free, happy

What I am doing (actions, behaviors): scooping dog poop. How I am being (feel, experiencing): irritated, disgusted, rushed.

In the illustrated examples it seems rational that our state of being is not a choice but a natural reaction to the circumstance or choice to 'do' certain things. Therefore if we are constantly being told that we have the power to choose what we do, but we believe that we have no control over how we will 'be', we may feel frantic to fill our lives with more doing.

We become desperate to make the 'right' choices to DO the 'right' things to experience the feelings we want in our lives. Makes sense right? When we've got a to-do list that makes us dread our day, add a trip to the nail salon, a phone date with the bestie, or maybe a pint of ice-cream. These 'things to look forward to' are the things we do in an attempt to experience the state of BEing that we crave.

This is obviously not totally a bad thing. Knowing we have the power to do certain things to feel the way we want. But it becomes a problem when we have zero capacity to do more.

Doing this will allow me to feel fulfilled. Doing that will allow me to become successful. Doing this to get ahead when I always feel behind. Doing that to find which direction I should go next. When we start with the doing, it becomes inevitable that no amount of doing is ever enough to fill us. When our doing always results in states of being that we cannot control, we feel hopeless to create the life we want.

DOING

RIDING A
FERRIS WHEEL

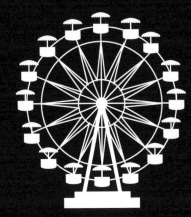

BEING
(FEELING, EXPERIENCING)

GIDDY, FREE,
HAPPY

DOING

SCOOPING
DOG POOP

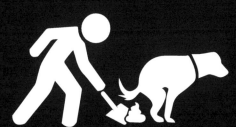

BEING
(FEELING, EXPERIENCING)

IRRITATED, RUSHED,
DISGUSTED

So, when we learn to consciously choose our state of being first, we very quickly create the life of joy, ease, and achievement that we have always dreamed of. Unfortunately, choosing into being can be more difficult at first, as it takes conscious awareness and lots of practice. Fortunately, though, it also creates results that we want and are more likely to enjoy.

Once we begin to see the distinction between approaching any circumstance from a place of doing vs. being, we begin creating the life that we love. Many of the strategies in this book are great tools to practice 'being' instead of 'doing' motherhood and life.

Let's pretend you are getting your little one ready for school. You see the steps in your head: this outfit, fix hair, shoes on, these bows... You are in doing mode. Even multitasking and getting stuff started in the house while you attempt to motivate your little one to focus and just stick to your to-do list! When suddenly you realize, your natural reaction to your circumstances is irritation, stress and the fear of being late-again.

Your 'beingness' is completely out of your control because you are so desperately focused on 'doing' the things you need to do to get out of the door on time and now, your child is having a meltdown. As soon as you realize that your state of 'being' is reactionary, you take a quick minute to remember that you can choose to 'be' yourself as a mom, instead of 'doing' motherhood. Remember, Mom WHO you are, utilize your genius and core values, receive her, get funcomfortable, be a flailure (yes, I said 'flail'. This jewel is coming up in part 7)! You tap into your core genius values of (let's say they are Movement, Laughter, and Connection) and allow yourself to be– even if it's only for just a moment. If I allow myself to just 'be'-- what would I 'do' differently?

And suddenly, with that simple practice, handfuls of new strategies and possible ways of 'doing' pop into your mind that you hadn't thought of before. And best of all, you begin to experience feelings you are more likely to enjoy like pride, motivation, and love.

What effect would that shift have on your morning? On getting out of the house on time? On your relationship with your child? On the way you see yourself as a mother and your confidence that you can do and be more next time? How magical might it make you feel in your mediocrity?

Do Less

DOING LESS IN YOUR life starts with one simple step. Assessing where you are wasting your time. If you take every single area of your life and the big goals you have in those things, about 20% of your efforts are producing 100% of your results. The other 80%? Balderdash! Nonsense! Prattle. Ok. Ok. I'm just kidding. Some of that 80% you spend your time doing simply because it's fun, or you enjoy it, or maybe these activities are things that are just not that difficult for you. How many things do you do that you sometimes think, I'm sure someone else could do this but I'm just gonna get it done real quick. Master mediocre mothers experience more ease, more joy, more presence because they have mastered the art of not doing crap anymore. Delegation, do it quicks, and do it nevers.

I use a simple chart called my *Delegation Map* (find a downloadable copy at www.mediocremommagic.com) in order to hash out my to-do list and get clear on what I can get off my list- asap. See the chart below. List out areas of your life at the top of rows, and create columns for

1. Tasks/To-Do

2. How do I feel when I think about this list?

3. What can I cross out? (do it never!)

4. What can I get done quickly?

5. What can I delegate? (Free+Hired)

Obviously, you know how to make a list of your to-dos. I like to separate the areas of my life into topics such as 'Kids School', 'Finances', 'Kids Sports', 'House Management', 'Health/Fitness', etc (we really do wear a dozen hats). Some categories such as Home Management or Your Business (if you own one) may need a *Delegation Map* of their own, to be broken down into smaller categories of home or business management. After making your to-do list in a category, the next step is always assessing how you feel once you look at the list. This is an important step because it will help you to decide which categories you will seek the most delegation support, and maybe even utilize funds to get paid help in those areas. If, when I look at the list of household management, and out of all of my lists I feel the most dread, fear and exhaustion (before I even do any of it!), I need to utilize my resources, financially and otherwise to get the most support for those tasks to get done asap. The emotional and time burden it lifts makes you abundantly available to get more things done by 'doing less' on your other lists as well.

Do-It Nevers

I want to begin with the most important of all. Just freaking saying no. To others and to yourself. The idea behind a Do it Never list is to identify tasks that are not creating results, as well as habits or behaviors that are not serving you well, and to intentionally avoid them in order to live a more fulfilling and productive life. By focusing on what not to do, you can create more space for the things that truly matter to you.

Quick Fix

Moving down to the quick wins, the tasks that take two seconds and give you an instant sense of accomplishment. You know what I'm talking about, lady! That pile of laundry? Toss it in the machine, throw in some soap, and boom, you're already one item down on that to-do list. That pile of dishes in the sink? Grab a sponge, scrub 'em down, and relish in the satisfaction of seeing that check mark on your list. Make it a luxury by popping in your headphones, tell your kids it's me time and catch up on your 'reading'.

And let's not forget about those easy errands, mama. Need to grab some milk and bread from the store? Don't put it off, put it in your online shopping cart, and check out now- or later! Maybe you've been meaning to send that birthday card to your sister-in-law. Well, go ahead and write out a magically mediocre ditty and pop it in the mail! Another one bites the dust.

Now, I know what you might be thinking. 'But Tessa, these are such small tasks, they won't make a dent in my never-ending to-do list!' Oh, but honey, that's where you're wrong. By starting with the easy stuff, you build momentum and motivation. You get that boost of confidence that comes from ticking off those small tasks, and suddenly that big project or daunting task doesn't seem so insurmountable.

Delegation

We've been conditioned to think that we have to do everything ourselves, that we are somehow failing if we can't handle it all. But Y'all, mediocre moms know that's just a big 'ol lie. You don't have to be Supermom. You don't have to do it all. Delegation is one of the master mediocre mamas most magical masteries.

"Mirror-cles"

THE 'PERFECT' MOTHER? OH she's over there, a master at the art of casting a vision for the future. And while I am so down with the crafty, create-your-world-fun of vision boards, daily dream bod and vacay visualizations, the most magical mediocre mother masters the powerful practice of rear-view visoning. When we utilize what has passed to cast a vision for what will come with no shame we become unstoppable mediocre dream magnets! As we continue the practice of rear-view visioning (creating a vision of who we want to be, what we want to feel, and what we want to do in the future based on assessing the past) we become more vulnerable and intimate with our desires and that makes this process more and more powerful.

First, let's talk mirror-cles. Not just miracles! Knowing what is coming is one of the most powerful tools we have as a mother. And, even better than knowing what is coming. Being prepared for what is coming (there is a difference). What is a Mirror-cle? Well, it's a manifestation of the power of forethought. For most of us mothers, having forethought for how we want some type of situation to go, requires first becoming aware of how a previously similar situation played out, and what we did not enjoy about it. A 'mirror-cle' is a Miracle that uses this nifty little proven scientific brain process known as the law of the mirror. What is the law of the mirror?

Ok so get this- The 'law of the mirror' refers to the discovery of mirror neurons in monkeys by some Italian neuroscientists in the 1990s.[7] Mirror neurons are a type of neuron that fires both when an animal performs an action and when the animal observes the same action being performed by another animal. So basically, our brain does not differentiate between doing something ourselves, or seeing someone else doing something (either in person or on a screen!) These mirror neurons explain why we experience anxiety while watching a thriller film, elation when that singer gets the gold buzzer on that talent competition, and even why we may get queasy watching someone else throw up.

Gnarly right? The discovery of mirror neurons is like discovering the secret sauce to create joy in your life as a mom. These little brain cells are the key to understanding how to utilize emotional contagion to create the energy we want to fill our homes, and to be the mom we always dreamed of. If you want your kids to be empathetic you must be an empathetic role model. Feels like a lot of pressure right? What if I told you in order to be it, we just have to see it. Immersing ourselves in the types of being we want to embody, increases our abilities to be that way with ease. By watching someone practice

VISIONING

6. REAR VIEW

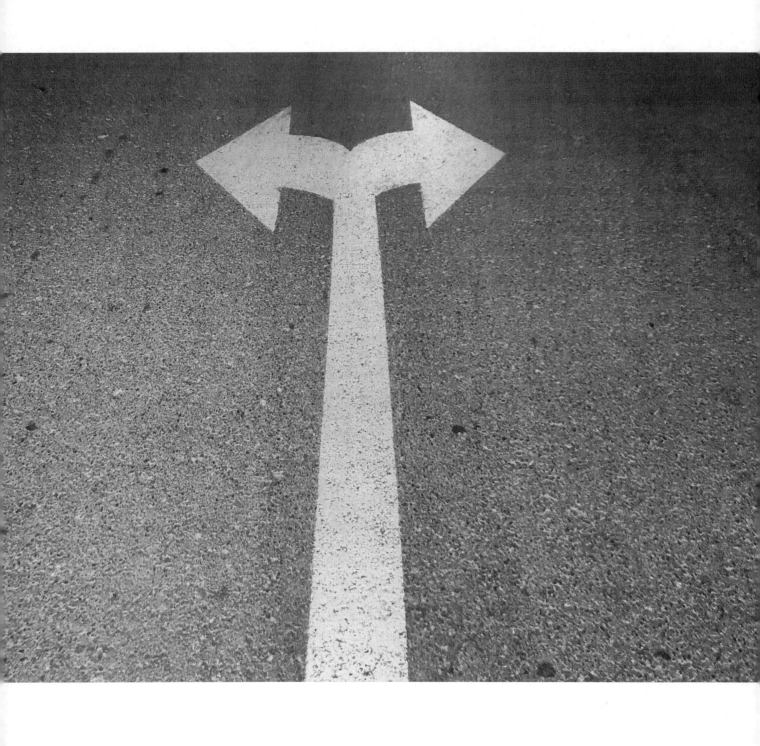

Decision Fatigue

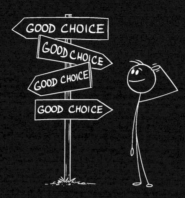

Life with Non-Negotiables

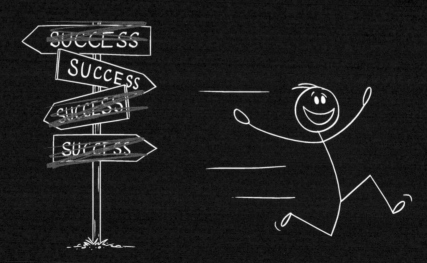

Decide Less

ARE YOU FEELING OVERWHELMED and exhausted from making decisions all day long? I totally get it - it's tough to keep up with the constant stream of choices we face as moms. You know what two things have made a huge difference in combating decision fatigue for me? Creating non-negotiables and deciding what you won't do.

Now, you might be thinking - 'What the heck are non-negotiables?' Well, my friend, they're basically things that you've decided are non-negotiable in your life. These are the things that are important to you, that you don't want to compromise on, no matter what.When you create non-negotiables, you take a whole bunch of decisions off the table. You don't have to waste precious mental energy deciding whether or not you should do something, because you already know that it's a non-negotiable. It's a decision you've already made, and you can move on to more important things.

And the best part? You can create non-negotiables anywhere in your life. They can be things like always eating dinner as a family, prioritizing self-care, or even something as simple as always making your bed in the morning. When you set these non-negotiables, you're freeing up mental space and energy to focus on the things that really matter.

Next, decide what you won't do. Yes, you read that right - sometimes, it's just as important to know what you won't do as it is to know what you will do.Think about it - when you have a whole bunch of options in front of you, it can be super overwhelming to decide what to do. But when you know what you're not willing to do, you can eliminate a whole bunch of choices and make things a lot easier on yourself.

For example, maybe you know that you won't compromise on your kids' bedtime routine. Or that you won't take on any new projects at work until you finish the ones you're already working on. When you know what you won't do, it frees up mental space and makes it easier to make decisions about what you will do. So, my dear mama, take some time to think about the things you won't do. They can be big or small, serious or silly - it doesn't matter. What matters is that you're taking some of the decision-making pressure off yourself. And don't forget to give yourself some love and grace along the way. You're doing an amazing job, even when it feels like the decisions never end.

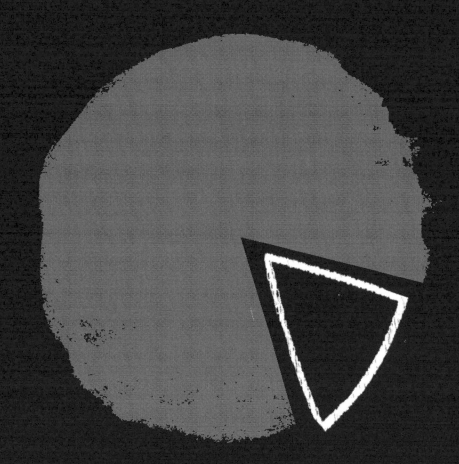

WASTE OF TIME   WORTH YOUR TIME

Alright, my fellow mama, let's cut to the chase. Yeah, you could spend hours scouring the internet for tips on what to delegate, who can take things off your plate, and how much it'll cost you. But let's be real, that's just a bunch of noise. You know why? Because you're not gonna do it, am I right?

Trust me, I know the feeling. Ten years ago, I was just like you. A trying-to-be-perfectionist who thought doing everything herself was easier than getting help. But here's the thing, mama. It's not easier. It's just making your life more stressful and overwhelming.

So, instead of wasting your time with all those webinars and podcasts, let me break it down for you. Look at your to-do list, and ask yourself, 'Can someone else do this for me?' The answer is probably yes. And guess what? It doesn't have to be expensive.

Maybe you can swap babysitting with a friend, or ask your partner or one of your kids to take care of dinner one night a week. And let's not forget about the power of good ol' fashioned bartering. Need help with something? Offer up your skills or services in exchange for theirs. It's a win-win situation. Checking in with the areas of life that are adding the most emotional weight, as you assessed, and utilize funds or bartering for those things that would be the greatest relief to get done without you. Let's take a load off, lady. And while we're at it- we're gonna go smash some decision fatigue. Oh yes...

patience, empathy, presence, it is not just the tools or strategies that we learn from that person, it is your state of being that changes. Like magic.

Almost a decade ago I was in the midst of a battle. From the outside, it may have seemed that the battle was between myself and my highly intelligent, iron willed 4 year old, but the true battle was within myself. Her intense emotions sent me into an emotional spiral. Frantically attempting to fix her so that my shot nerves and fragile spirit could get a rest. I read books, tried strategies that ran the gamut from redirection (never worked) to time out (she never stayed) to that one time I held her in near silence (reminding her she could get down when she was calm and that I loved her and she was safe) in my arms as she raged and flailed for 2 hours. Now, I am not saying the dozens of strategies I read about and tried wouldn't have worked, only that they did not. And the reason why they didn't? Me.

Until I used the mirror. Now, I honestly cannot tell you why or how I figured out to attempt this strategy but it was a profound blessing.

What you are experiencing

What you are visualizing

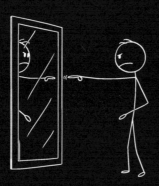 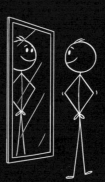

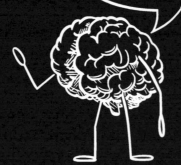

How to Rear View Vision Your Triggers:

During this time of our lives I knew that her big feelings and me getting triggered were almost a given for any day. So, not only did I know what was coming, I decided to prepare. As if I were going daily into battle. I began to spend time every single morning visioning her in her uncontrollable rage. The one that made me an emotional mess and I could not stop. And instead of visualizing how I would fix the problem, what I would say, what I would do, I envisioned myself with her as she raged and I saw myself being calm.

I visualized long enough (maybe 2-3 minutes tops) until I felt that calm permeate my body and even while visualizing this moment that was so triggering to me emotionally, I was completely calm and at peace. And do you know what happened? I was calm. Not sad, not scared, not feeling like I was failing.

Finally, my soul was at rest. In those moments I was clear, and I honestly cannot tell you what strategies I employed that every single day distracted her, supported her, cheered her up, or diffused the issue with ease. All I know is that It was working. That was all I needed. To vision with a rear-view and focus on how I wanted to Be.

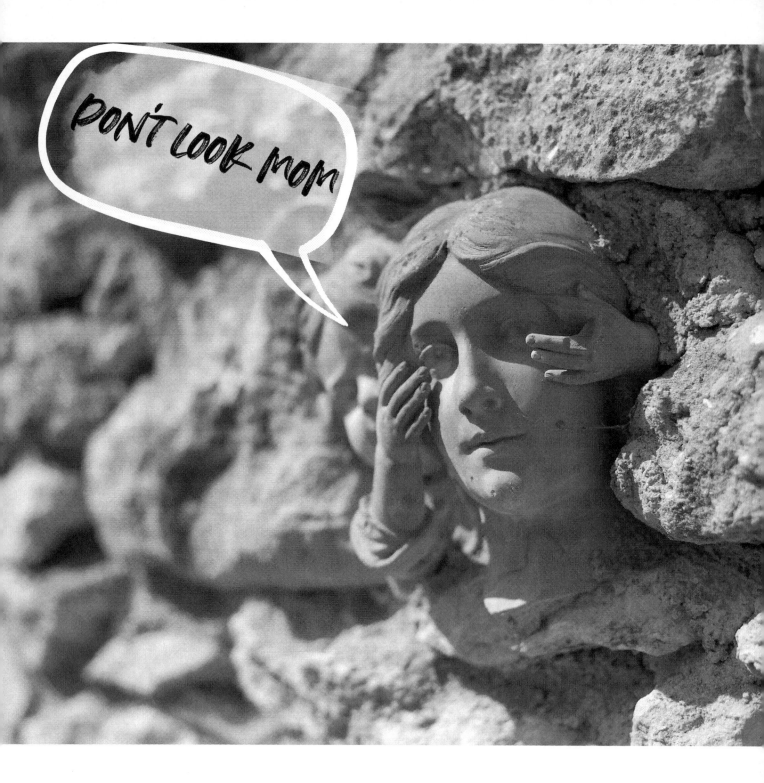

Your Shadow

REMEMBER PETER PAN'S SHADOW? How it was a nasty little menace, but also his best friend? He couldn't imagine his life without it?

When we hear talk about 'healing your shadow,' what it means is exploring and addressing the parts of ourselves that we try to hide or ignore. You know, the parts of us that we're not exactly proud of, like our insecurities, fears, and negative thought patterns. It's kind of like cleaning out the closet you've been avoiding—sometimes it can get way messier before it's put right again, but it's so worth it in the end!

By facing these parts of ourselves and working through them, we can gain a deeper understanding and acceptance of who we are. This can lead to more fulfilling relationships, a stronger sense of self, and a more authentic life. Heck ya! Sign me up for that!

I've been trying to hide from my fear of my own underperformance, my own mediocrity, my entire life. Owning this 'shadow' part of ourselves is claiming it as a friend, embracing and leveraging our own negative beliefs about ourselves for our own growth. Instead of continuing our lifelong coverup and avoidance. Because how has that been working so far? (((Ever heard the saying, what we resist, persists?)))

This entire book is an exercise in exposing, owning and befriending my shadow. It's not about a self-deprecating ownership of our flaws, or even trying to fix them. It's about unearthing the underlying beliefs that create all of the other garbage that prevents us from believing that the magic is in the ordinary. The underlying false identity that lies to us and tells us that we can't be 'extra' if we are not 'enough'.

I shouldn't run if I can't run fast. I cannot be happy if my child is sad. I should not bake if my cookies are not the best. If I try to create the relationships and gatherings I crave, I will be rejected. If I tell my husband I want this, he will laugh at me. I shouldn't attempt surfing if I'm worse than everyone out there. I will look dumb. Even though my soul craves to be one with the sea. I should not attempt dancing because I will look like a floppy idiot. Even though my heart yearns to be silly and free with my friends.

Owning your shadow is:

Becoming the most stoked, worst surfer. Becoming the best, worst dancer than ever stepped foot on that dance floor. Doing things because your heart craves them, in spite of your shadow. That's how we become friends with our darkest parts. And eventually, maybe even gain freedom from them.

If we believe the things that our shadow tells us about our Mediocrity, all we can be is limited.

If we make it our friend, we inevitably become limitless.

RESISTING YOUR SHADOW

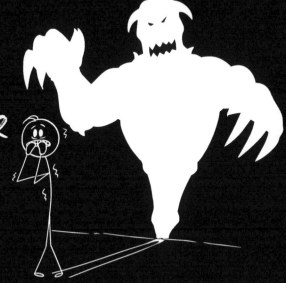

BEFRIENDING YOUR SHADOW

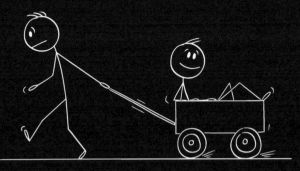

FUN
7. UN COMF

ORTABLE

MORE FUN

I like playing with that space between
laughter and discomfort where your
discomfort can also make you laugh, and
you're confused about the mixed feelings.
That's challenging, and I think that's what
makes for some of the best art.

-Hari Kondabolu[2]

ARE YOU READY FOR the wild sense of freedom and possibility that makes moms the most magicallist of all? It's time to embrace the power of getting funcomfortable, y'all. Funcomfortable- while not a word I coined by any means— is the essence of my being. It's my most favorite mediocre magic principle of all. And something I firmly believe can be tapped into and magnified by every single human being on this planet. What the crap is it? Well, getting Funcomfortable is all about pushing yourself out of your comfort zone and doing things that might make you feel a bit nervous or scared, but in the process of doing them, bring you joy, fulfillment and growth.

Ok... so I hear you. You're wondering, *how can adding more discomfort to my life allow me to experience more joy and ease in my motherhood?* Well, here's the thing, it's not about adding more discomfort. It's about adding more *fun* to your discomfort. Discomfort is a given. Pain is not optional in life. But suffering is. And if there's anything my personal experience has taught me it's that the most powerful way to tell suffering to suck it, is to intentionally make anything uncomfortable, painful, freaking sucky– fun. Not surprisingly, myriads of studies have shown that people who regularly engage in activities that make them feel anxious or nervous report higher levels of life satisfaction and happiness over time. Not a shocker to this girl here who in college ran down our street in glow in the dark Cat face underwear on Halloween. Like, I get that I'm crazy, but anyone- introvert, extrovert, can leverage (in much more subtle ways) the power of Funcomfortable. Cuz who doesn't want more happiness in their life?

When we become moms, we often get so caught up in the day-to-day responsibilities that we forget to have fun. We forget to take risks, to challenge ourselves, and to do things that make us feel alive. But getting funcomfortable regularly can help bring joy, ease, and accomplishment to our lives.

So first the elephant in the room– Our comfort zones. Funcomfortable offers us a clean break– a way out when stayin' in the warm cozy familiar seems much more doable. As moms, we tend to stick to what we know because it feels safe and secure— and honestly, we've got enough other crap to worry about. But when we consciously choose to push ourselves out of our comfort zones and try something new, we become a more resilient, relaxed, joyful mother. And sometimes we can discover new passions, hobbies, and talents we never knew we had.

A few years ago, I was in a community of women who were all trying to build our businesses. At that time, I was focused on growing my coaching business and bringing in clients, while also trying to gain control over my family's finances and break free from the vicious cycle of living paycheck to paycheck and relying on debt.

As part of this community, I stumbled upon a fun money mindset challenge group that encouraged us to engage in uncomfortable activities on a daily basis. The first few days involved journaling and sharing our money patterns, examining how we were raised, and identifying our true desires. It was an incredibly powerful experience.

But it was the second-to-last day that truly blew me away. We were challenged to expand our monthly financial goals for our business by multiplying them by 100 and writing ourselves a fake check for that amount. To take things even further and really drive the visualization exercise home (remember, the law of the mirror), we were instructed to 'deposit' the money in a way that felt real to our brains.

Some chose to pretend to make a mobile deposit or 'give' the money to a spouse who would 'deposit' it in the bank. Others went to the bank and pretended to make the deposit, filling out a deposit slip and then heading home. But I wanted to take things a step further.

I drove to the bank and actually deposited the fake check with a real teller. My anxiety was through the roof - my heart was racing, my chest was tight, and my breathing was shallow. I even went live for the whole event in my Facebook group. I pushed through the discomfort pulsating in my throat, chest, down my arms, and explained to the teller that I was doing an exercise for a class and needed to 'deposit' the check and get a receipt.

There was some confusion at first, but once the teller and his coworkers understood what was going on, their eyes filled with enlightenment and joy. They laughed together, delighted by the absurdity and creativity of the exercise. The teller even returned my fake check with a handwritten receipt, complete with a smiley face. 'This made my day,' he said.

In that moment, something shifted within me. The anxiety and fear that had been coursing through my body suddenly transformed into exhilaration and joy. I felt a surge of power and strength throughout my entire body, as if I were unstoppable. The tension in my arms dissolved, replaced by a sense of unbridled energy that radiated all the way to my fingertips.

This incredible experience was one of the most funcomfortable things I've ever done, but it was also one of the most transformative. It taught me that pushing through discomfort and embracing the unknown can lead to incredible growth and empowerment. Doing it intentionally gave me back all power. And that anxiety, fear and tension can transform in an instant to the most potent excitement and enthusiasm I have ever experienced.

Just like I experienced at the bank, seeking funcomfortable experiences can also help us manage stress and anxiety. Centuries of great thinkers have leveraged this power of getting Funcomfortable with the powerful principles of Stoicism. You see, the ancient Greeks and Romans knew a thing or two about managing their emotions. And one technique they used was called negative visualization - and no, it's not as scary as it sounds!

Basically, they imagine the worst possible scenario in a given situation, and then prepare themselves to handle it. They utilize the imagined Funcomfortable experience to exercise their anxiety and shift into a more relaxed energy around something they fear. By visualizing the worst-case scenario, they take away some of the power that anxiety and fear have over you. By mentally preparing for the worst, they actually feel more confident and in control when the time comes. (Similar to my experience with my daughter's behavior in the last section).

My favorite part of the entire concept of getting FUNComfortable has to be the example we set when Funcomfortable becomes our way of life! Getting funcomfortable makes us powerful role models for our children. When we show our kids that we are willing to take risks and try new things, even when we are afraid, we're teaching them to be brave, confident, and adventurous. We're showing them that it's okay to fail and that it's important to do hard things.

So, how do you start? Dance around in your pajamas, do karaoke, ride a horse, get the freak up and sing karaoke at that party - whatever it is that makes you feel alive and maybe- terrified. Remember that discomfort does not have to equal suffering, and that getting out of your comfort zone can lead to personal growth, improved well-being, and a more joyful life.

And the best part? The benefits of getting funcomfortable spill over into every area of your life. When you feel more confident and capable, you approach challenges with greater ease and determination. You find joy and meaning in your daily activities, and you experience a greater sense of accomplishment and fulfillment in your personal and professional pursuits. BAM! So here's a fun little list of funcomfortable Double-Dog-Dares for ya. Trust me, sister, it will turn out so much better than you think.

Funcomfortable Dares

- Say 'over and out' after every sentence.
- Put on headphones at the park and dance-like no one is watching (cliche-but do it!)
- Go live on social media and sing
- Go live on social media —PERIOD
- Break-dance battle one of your kids
- Message 5 of your favorite Instagramers and ask them to write you back.
- Show all major life stages from birth through death in interpretive dance form.
- Let another person post a status on your behalf.

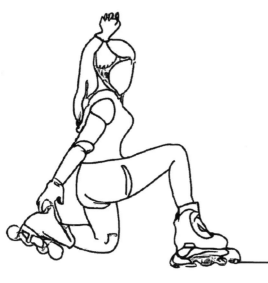

- Attempt to do a magic trick.
- Roller skate with tricks
- Rock climb some real rocks on a whim
- Karaoke at that party
- Photo scavenger hunt
- Play on the floor with your kids
- Talk to the first person you see when you leave your house
- Schedule a mermaid photo shoot
- Or Boudoir photo shoot
- Or just any freaking photos hoot of just you- for you

BE A FLAILURE

"

The sense of disequilibrium within our soul is actually what Sparks the most powerful action. That sucky feeling of being off-kilter or out of sync. It`s just like our arms flailing out when we're about to lose our balance. So, when we feel unmotivated, intentionally throwing off our balance with a Spark! of discomfort ignites the yummiest movement & momentum.

-Tessa Aranda

"

HOW TO BE A SURFER IN 5 STEPS

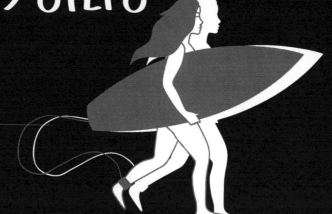

1. Look like a surfer
2. Get in the waves
3. Look like an idiot- flail
4. Learn your equilibrium and the rhythm of the water
5. Conquer a wave

THIS IS SO FLIPPIN' crucial. Don't skip it — k? Our problem with striving for perfection? It's not that we're afraid to fail, it's that we're afraid to flail. To be a beginner. To start where we suck when everyone else seems to have it all figured out. We're constantly comparing ourselves to other women, wondering how they're able to juggle so much and still make it look effortless. We ask them for tips and tricks, but when they start telling us about their own struggles and failures on the way to getting there, we shut down. We don't want to hear about the messy middle, we just want the shortcut to success.

But flailing is totally not something to be afraid of. In fact, it can become your best friend if you let it. See, the key to success is not avoiding failure, but embracing it. I'm sure you know this blah, blah, blah everyone talks about it. You attempt more shots, you'll make more baskets. Michael Jordan all that jazz. But if you look further, it's about being willing to try new things, even if it means starting at the bottom and looking like a complete beginner. And the more you're willing to be knocked off balance, the more you'll learn and grow.

I started surfing not even a year ago. (Well, for the first time in 15 years. I was never good, just did it a few times as a teen). When I started I went with a group of moms who switched off being in the water and watching kids. I was by far, the most pathetic member of the 'Mom's surf swap'. I could barely stay balanced on the board lying flat, struggled with my weak little arms to paddle out past the waves, and tumbled over the falls of huge waves in my lame attempts to catch them before they smashed me. I was definitely flailing.

But something changed in me a few months in, I stopped looking around and focusing on the head chatter about what all the other surfers must think about my flailing attempts, and I truly embraced my mediocrity. I started actually listening to the other moms when I would get out of the water when they would ask me 'Did you have fun?' Never once did they ask 'How did you do?' Yet I always over-explained how terrible I was and the play-by-play of how I was maybe getting better. After always hearing 'how fun was it'. Something started shifting in me. I started listening to them. I started looking for the fun. I stopped judging my experience on how much I flailed but instead, by how much I freaking rocked at having the best time ever with myself in my flailing. I tried crap that was embarrassing because I sucked so bad (like sitting on my board- y'all takes a minute for your core to learn that balance) and gut laughed with myself at my attempts. And to my surprise, I actually got so much better, stronger, and was figuring stuff out. And now, it's my favorite. I'm not just doing surfing anymore. I am a surfer.

Don't be afraid to start that new habit, set a new expectation, or pursue a new dream. Sure, you might fail at first. You might feel like a flailure. But that's freaking okay! That's kinda the point! Embrace the experience of it, and stay anchored in the magic that comes from upsetting your equilibrium. When you start to see the beauty in the messy middle, you'll find that flailing becomes a powerful tool for growth and transformation. And who knows, you might just surprise yourself with what you're capable of achieving. So get out there and flail like the bad-a mediocre mama you are!

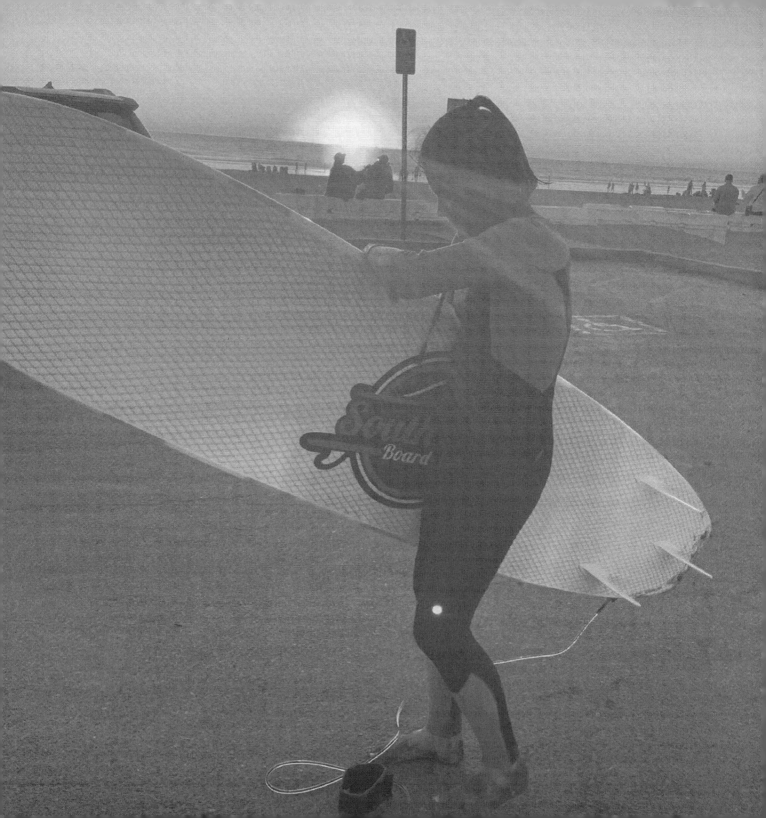

Intentionally Imperfect Daily

Are you tired of striving for perfection every day? This, for me, was where this all began. I was so sick of feeling like I was constantly falling short and getting stressed out about it. Like, ya, I'm going to fall short. Always. So like, how can we shift this? Well, I've got some good news for you: it's time to embrace the power of intentionally being imperfect, baby!

Here's the deal: we're all human and we all make mistakes. But instead of letting those mistakes get us down, we can choose to celebrate them as opportunities to learn, grow, and have a little fun along the way. Think about it - how many times have you accidentally burned the dinner, or forgotten to pack your kid's lunch? It happens to the best of us! But when we approach these moments with a sense of playfulness and curiosity, rather than shame and frustration, we open ourselves up to a world of possibilities.

Let's take it a step further, though. When we choose to be *intentionally* imperfect, we give ourselves permission to try new things, take risks, and step outside of our comfort zones. We can let go of the fear of failure and embrace the excitement of the unknown. And when we inevitably stumble, we can dust ourselves off, learn from our mistakes, and keep moving forward. Because doing it imperfectly was the point. Too often, we hang too many expectations on our attempts, our experiences, our whole flippin life. This book for example, could have been a big, huge, gigantic deal. I have wanted to write and publish a book my entire life. If I hung my hat on my first attempt being the deal breaker, the magic creation that got me on Good Morning America, Drew Barrymore's couch (cuz Oprah doesn't have a show anymore right? Plus I like Drew better anyway.)

Do you know how frozen I would have been? Can you imagine how stressful the process, how many more years it would have taken to get this incredible life changing work that I am so passionate about out into the world? If it had to be Oprah level perfect? Discoverable? One hit wonder worthy!?!? I hope my making a choice to finally get it all organized and into your hands in less than 60 days is a divine example of imperfect action in, uh, action. I hope whatever typos, run-ons and weird stories... are an experiential example of every single word I am typing. Every principle I cling to. Magic that is done and shared. Is one hundred times better than perfect. And infinitely better than magic that is never shared at all.

Here's the real kicker: intentionally being imperfect actually leads to greater success and happiness in the long run. When we release the pressure to be perfect, we free up our mental and emotional energy to focus on the things that truly matter - our relationships, our passions, and our own sense of well-being.

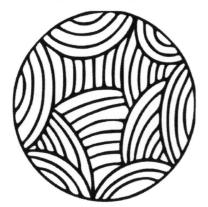

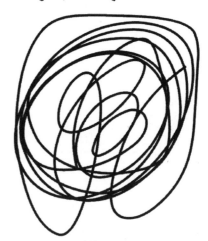

INTENTIONALLY imperfect
- REFLECTIVE
- INNOVATIVE
- GROWTH FOCUSED
- HOPEFUL
- CONTENT
- LET'S GO EASILY

ACCIDENTALLY imperfect
- RIGID
- ASHAMED
- REGRETFUL
- RESENTFUL
- PROJECTING EMOTIONS

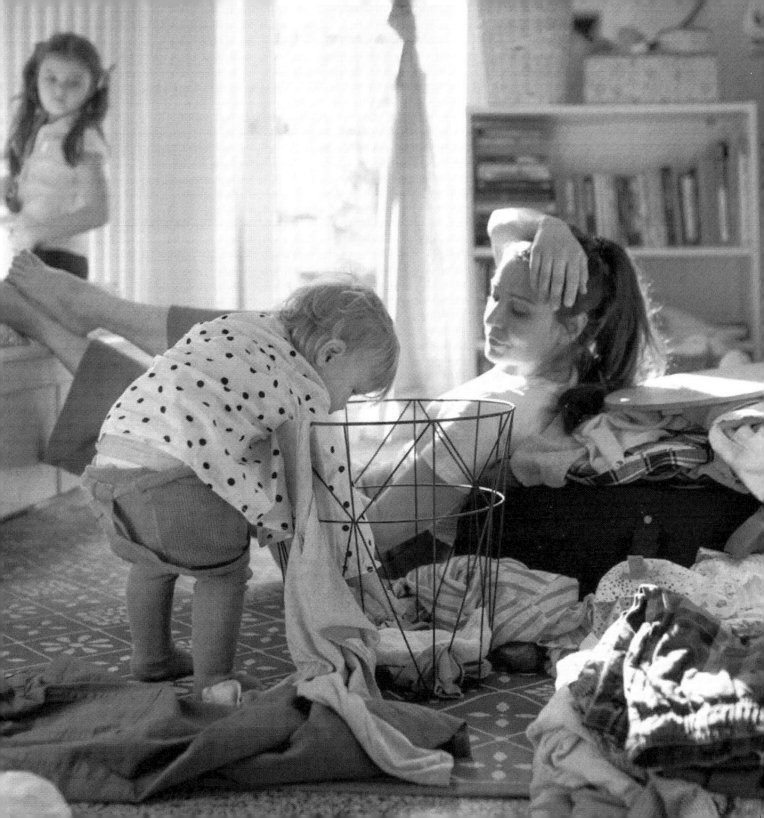

When we try to be perfect, we put a lot of pressure on ourselves. We get anxious and stressed out, and we're constantly worried about making mistakes. But when we choose to be imperfect, we take the pressure off ourselves. We give ourselves permission to make mistakes and to learn from them.

We're going to make mistakes no matter what. It's inevitable. But when we choose to be intentionally imperfect, we take control of the situation. We're not reacting to our mistakes; we're choosing them. And that can be insanely empowering. When we choose to be intentionally imperfect, we're also modeling a healthy attitude for our children. We're showing them that it's okay to make mistakes, that it's part of the learning process. We're teaching them that perfection isn't the goal; growth is.

So how do we choose to be intentionally imperfect? Here are a few ideas:

Try something new. When we try something new, we're almost guaranteed to make mistakes. But if we go into it with the expectation that we're going to be imperfect, we can enjoy the process more. We can learn from our mistakes and grow as a person.

Embrace the messy. Life is messy, especially when you have kids. Instead of trying to control everything and keep it all neat and tidy, embrace the chaos. Let your kids make messes (within reason, of course), and don't stress about the state of your house. Life is too short to worry about every little thing.

Be vulnerable. It's easy to try to present a perfect image to the world, but that's not authentic. When we're vulnerable and show our imperfections, we connect with others on a deeper level. We show that we're human, and we create space for others to be imperfect too.

Practice self-compassion. When we make mistakes, it's easy to beat ourselves up about it. But self-compassion is key. Treat yourself with the same kindness and understanding that you would show a good friend. Remember that mistakes are part of the process, and that you're doing the best you can.

Choosing to be intentionally imperfect isn't always easy. We live in a culture that values perfection, and it can be hard to go against the grain. But when we choose to be imperfect, we're giving ourselves the gift of freedom. We're allowing ourselves to make mistakes and learn from them. We're embracing the messiness of life and modeling a healthy attitude for our children. And that's pretty powerful.

How to Be "Intentionally Imperfect"

1. TRY NEW STUFF

2. EMBRACE MESS

3. BE VULNERABLE

4. PRACTICE SELF- COMAPSSION

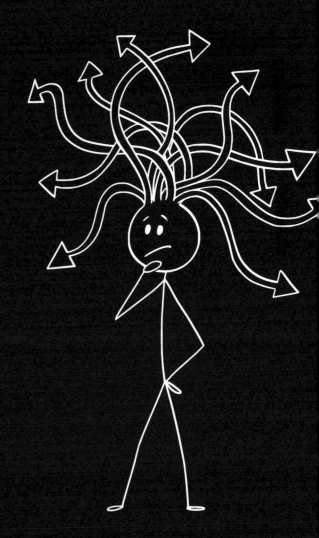

8. BiG

FUN

Giant Leaps For Woman-Kind

How can we set and smash big goals from a place of ease & wonder? Are you ready to have some big fun in your life? I'm not talking about just the usual daily tasks, but about making some big leaps towards the life you want. You know, the one where you wake up feeling energized and excited about what's in store for the day, and not just trying to survive until bedtime. Are you tired of feeling like you're just going through the motions, constantly running on autopilot, and barely keeping your head above water? It's time to take a quantum leap and create some big fun in your life.

Now, when I say 'big fun,' I don't just mean going on a vacation or having a spa day (although those things can be fun too). I'm talking about making major changes in your life that bring you joy, ease, and fulfillment.

Big fun could mean setting a big, audacious goal that scares you a little (or a lot). Maybe you want to start your own business, run a marathon, write a book, or learn a new skill that you've always been curious about. Whatever it is, it should be something that excites you and pushes you out of your comfort zone.

It could also mean making big changes to your daily routine to create more joy and ease. Maybe you've been feeling overwhelmed and burnt out, so you decide to hire a nanny to help with the kids a few days a week. Or you start waking up earlier to have some quiet time to yourself before the chaos of the day begins. Or you start saying 'no' to commitments that don't align with your values and priorities.

The key is to identify what would bring you the most joy and fulfillment, and then take action to make it happen. And here's the thing: taking a quantum leap doesn't have to be scary or overwhelming. In fact, it can be incredibly empowering and exciting.

Here are a few examples of big fun that moms have taken in their own lives:

One mom decided to leave her corporate job and start a business selling organic baby food. She had always been passionate about healthy eating and had a knack for cooking, so she decided to turn that passion into a career. It wasn't easy, but she was able to build a successful business that allowed her to spend more time with her family and do work that she truly loved.

Another mom had always dreamed of running a marathon, but had never been much of a runner. She decided to sign up for a beginner's running group and started training for the race. It was tough at first, but she stuck with it and eventually completed the marathon. Not only did she feel incredibly proud of herself, but she also developed a love for running and continued to do it regularly.

A third mom was feeling overwhelmed and burnt out from juggling work and family responsibilities. She decided to hire a part-time nanny to help with the kids a few days a week, which allowed her to have some much-needed downtime to recharge and focus on her own needs. It was a big decision, but it made a huge difference in her overall well-being and quality of life.

Here's the thing: we often think that the only way to achieve our big goals is by taking small, incremental steps. When we believe it will take us three years to accomplish a goal like buying a house, moving across the country, creating that children's program you've been dreaming of, etc. it will take three years. It may even continue to take three years over and over again.Suddenly a decade is past and you wonder if that leap will ever come. But when we set a date and decide, *this will be done in 6 months*, you see new possibilities and take much different actions. The result may take eight, but compared to your original belief that it would take 3 years, you took a significantly bigger leap and got it done almost 2 years ahead of your original schedule. That's the power of big fun magic in action.

It's all about changing your mindset and taking a big fun approach. Instead of just taking baby steps towards your goals, ask yourself: what would be the most fun way to make a big leap towards my goal? The biggest leaps we ever take are leaps in our belief. After we choose to believe that something is possible for us, and make a decision to take just one step in that direction, you'll find that you have more creativity and inspiration to make those leaps. You might even surprise yourself with what you can accomplish!

The trick is to not worry if you don't know exactly how to get there yet. When you set a big fun goal, the path will start to reveal itself. You'll start to attract the resources, ideas, and people you need to make it happen.

So, whether it's starting your own business, running a marathon, or learning a new skill, take a big fun approach. Set a big goal, and let the excitement and joy guide you on the journey towards achieving it. What is a Big Fun Dream or Goal that you have? Want to take a leap? Write it out, and decide to drastically shorten your timeline. Give yourself some time to sit with it and observe, what becomes possible? What creative inspiration floods in? Take note, and act.

EATING THE FROG

OH GIRL, GET READY to make some waves! It's time to shake things up and create some big fun in our lives! You know those goals that seem big, intimidating, and impossible to avoid? Yep. We're talking about the ones that make you want to crawl back into bed and hide under the covers. Guess what? It's time to take a stand and eat that frog!

Eating the frog is an expression that the internet cannot figure out the origin of. In Brian Tracy's 2001 hit book, "Eat That Frog!: 21 Great Ways to Stop Procrastinating and Get More Done in Less Time" He attributes the quote to Mark Twain, but there is no evidence it was him, and is attributed to many different authors. Anyway, Tracy used the phrase to describe the idea of tackling the most important, and often the most dreaded, task on your to-do list first thing in the morning. The belief is that if you start your day by getting the most difficult task out of the way, it sets a positive tone for the rest of your day and eliminates any stress or anxiety associated with having that gruesome task hanging over your head. Twain was misquoted to have said, 'if the first thing you do in the morning is eat a live frog, nothing worse will happen to you for the rest of the day'. It's a good quote though right? Similarly , if you start your day by accomplishing the biggest and most challenging task, it'll be uphill from there and you'll feel more productive, confident and in control. The twinkling light in the distance will appear so much brighter. Thinking about eating the frog is most often worse than actually eating the frog.

So how do we get clear on exactly what those big things are? Those 'frogs' in our day and in this season of life? But let's be real - as moms, how often do we wish someone would just tell us what is the most important task that will move the needle forward on our goals and our stress levels? The problem is when we attack all that needs to be done without forethought, we end up feeling like everything is the frog. It's overwhelming and makes us want to throw in the towel before we even start.

That's why we need to break it down into two simple steps: first, figure out what the frog is, and second, just eat the damn frog. Sounds simple enough, right? But too often, we're told to 'just do it' without any guidance on what 'it' is.

So many women I have worked with have expressed to me this frustration. For most of us, having been raised in the public school system (not learning to trust our own spirit, but to obey a delegation) our familiarity with the decision making skills that the real world expects of us is a foreign language.

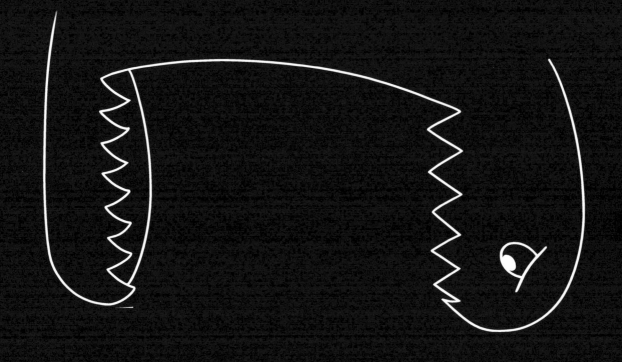
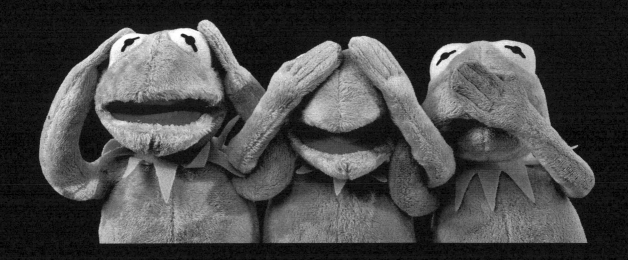

What are the tasks that will move the needle and create the most space in our lives? In the work environment, the job of your boss, of course, is to delegate what you need to get done, how and when to do them and to prioritize your tasks. Since one's 'Boss' does not exist in a family circle, as a mom, how much of your day is spent wishing there was someone who would identify your day's most important task and prioritize the rest of the day's activities. What will move the needle forward the most on our myriad of goals while experiencing minimal stress and allow you just a moment to sit back, enjoy and be in the present?

I don't believe that mothers have a hard time doing hard stuff. We do difficult things every day because we have to - like changing a dirty diaper or cleaning up a mess. *Did I want to change that diaper? No.* Eat the frog. *Just do it.* Countless times we have procrastinated the changing of a poop, creating more misery as we contemplated actually getting it done. *Will it stink? Will my baby whine and scream? Will the poop 'somehow' end up smeared on the walls?*

We know the mental and emotional weight of these questions and of a delay. So we have learned. Just do it. But when it comes to tackling bigger goals and tasks, we can feel paralyzed because we don't know where to start. Each task feels like the most dreadful, most important, most overwhelming and most urgent.

So, before we can utilize tools like accountability, motivation, or inspiration, we need to get clear on ONE frog. When we are not clear on the one 'frog' in our day, we experience discomfort and frustration thinking about eating all the frogs and then becoming paralyzed (because eating 20 frogs a day doesn't even seem human). Then, we go sit on the couch and scroll. When we are not clear on the one 'frog' for this season of our life, we feel listless, bored, uninspired, stuck, and possibly even resentful or depressed.

We need to identify the most important goals that will move the needle forward and create more ease, flow, and joy in our lives. So let's eat that frog, one bite at a time, and watch as the rest falls into place with ease and confidence. Are you ready to take the first bite?

So, moms, what's your big fun? What's the thing that would bring you the most joy and fulfillment, even if it feels scary or overwhelming at first? Take some time to reflect on this, and then take action to make it happen. You deserve to live a life filled with big fun, and you have the power to make it a reality.

What can you do now? Make a list of the 'Big Fun' goals you have for your family, yourself, or your home. Which one thing would change everything? Create space for you to create the other goals with joy and ease? Allow time and space through journaling or meditation to receive an answer that you might not expect, or maybe one you knew all along. Give yourself permission to focus only on that one thing. Imagine and vision your perfect world around this goal. Delegate this 'thing' as your '#1 job' for the time being, until a big shift occurs. Give yourself permission to relax and release the other 'frogs' with trust that your focus will yield results in all areas of your life. If you are already focused and committed to your big life-changing frog for right now, take time to vision, write and recommit to your end vision. And to believe that even faster and bigger leaps are possible.

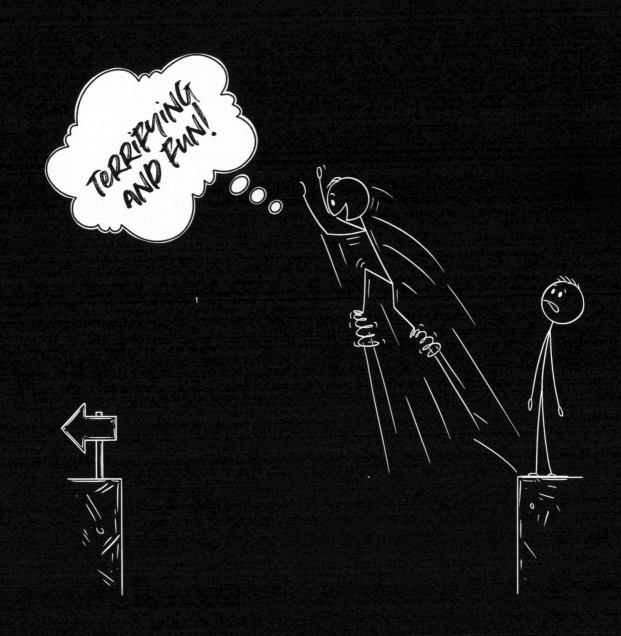

Movement vs. Momentum

IT'S TIME FOR A little reality check. We all know that making big changes can be tough. And I'm not talking about just throwing a few bucks around here and there. I'm talking about those huge, life-changing decisions like moving across the country or putting your kids in school. The kind of stuff that seems impossible until it magically falls into place at the very last second.

Now, here's the deal. There's a big difference between movement and momentum. Movement can be all over the place, erratic, and not really getting you anywhere. But momentum, oh baby, that's when things start really picking up speed. When you've got momentum on your side, you're not just moving, you're flying towards your goals at lightning speed. This means identifying the things that bring joy and ease to their family and making them a regular part of their routine. It also means being willing to let go of things that aren't working and trying something new.

One way to start is by taking small, consistent steps towards their goals. For example, if a mom wants to create a more peaceful and organized home, she can start by setting aside 10 minutes each day to declutter and tidy up. By doing this consistently, she will create momentum towards her goal and eventually create a home that brings her joy and ease.

But consistency is not all you need, a lot of people think that if they just keep doing the same thing over and over again, success is bound to come knocking on their door eventually. But that's a load of baloney. You need more than just consistency, you need momentum. And that's when things get really exciting.

Let me give you an example. A couple of years ago, I was working on my coaching program and I was doing all the right things. I was posting every day, connecting with those who needed my services, building relationships, and I knew my message inside and out. But I still wasn't getting the kind of traction I wanted. I was moving, but I wasn't gaining any momentum.

So, I decided to shake things up. I told my community to post a picture of themselves holding a sign with their goals on it, and I promised to create something special for them. And then, bam! Momentum hit me like a ton of bricks. My community was buzzing with excitement, and I ended up making 14 sales calls in one week, with 7 of them signing up for my coaching program.

Now, even if you do not own a business, the moral of the story, mamas, is that momentum can be created in an instant, but it has to be a game-changer. It's not just about consistency, it's about finding that leverage point that really gets people excited and moving towards their goals. Trying different, creative approaches to the same problem while maintaining consistency. Take a look at your life and ask yourself, are you just moving, or are you building momentum? Trust me, the distinction is huge, and it can make all the difference in creating the joyful, easy life you want for yourself and your family.

As a mom who struggled for years with postpartum depression when my kids were so young, this principle has been key to building the type of relationships I want with my oldest three kids especially. For years, I battled with depression, frustration, resentment, and reactivity. After finally receiving a diagnosis and the help I needed, my behaviors slowly started to change, but, unfortunately, my kids' brains did not. All of the neural pathways that my kids developed to not trust my reactions, to be unsure of being heard and supported in our home, needed more than my consistency in behaving differently in order to be rewired.

I was creating a movement for more gentle interactions, more support and compassion and connection in our home, but I struggled for a couple years to find those leverage points where we would finally find the momentum forward I craved. Trust was building slowly, but being completely different as a family felt so far out of reach.

Until I did some things that were drastically different in attempts to gain traction, and create that momentum of hope, healing, and harmony in our home. (2 years of coaching utilizing the Gibson Banning method, energy and emotional healing modalities, and learning to apply the atonement of Jesus Christ were those things for me).

So let's dig deeper for a minute into the difference between movement and momentum. Movement is all well and good, but it doesn't always get us where we want to go. We can be moving a million miles a minute, checking things off our to-do list left and right, and yet still feel like we're not making any real progress toward our goals. We might feel scattered, unfocused, and like we're just spinning our wheels.

Momentum, on the other hand, is a game-changer. When we have momentum on our side, we're not just moving, we're moving with intention and purpose. We're focused, we're driven, and we're making steady progress toward our goals. We're like a rolling ball, picking up speed and power as we go, and nothing can stop us.

So, how can we as moms create momentum in our lives? It starts with getting clear on what we really want and setting some specific, achievable goals. It means identifying the actions that will move us toward those goals and committing to taking those actions consistently, day in and day out. Being open to discovering and leveraging new possible strategies while consistently maintaining the things that are working.

For example, if your goal is to have a more peaceful and harmonious household, you might identify some specific actions that will help you get there. Maybe it's spending 10 minutes each day in quiet reflection, setting clear boundaries with your family, or making time for regular family meetings. Whatever it is, make a plan and stick to it.

As you take these actions consistently, you'll start to build momentum. You'll feel more confident, more in control, and more aligned with your values and goals. And as you continue to build momentum, you'll find that it gets easier and easier to keep moving forward. Leverage becomes inevitable as we seek inspiration possibilities with our sights on the things we really want, committing to taking intentional, purposeful action every day. With momentum on our side, we can achieve anything we set our minds to and create more joy and ease in our families.

Do you currently have an area of your life where you feel like you're constantly pushing and striving, but not really seeing progress? Now, when do you feel the most energized and alive in your day to day life? What activity or task is usually involved during those moments? Is there any way you can integrate the two? This is a powerful practice to meditate on and journal for this principle.

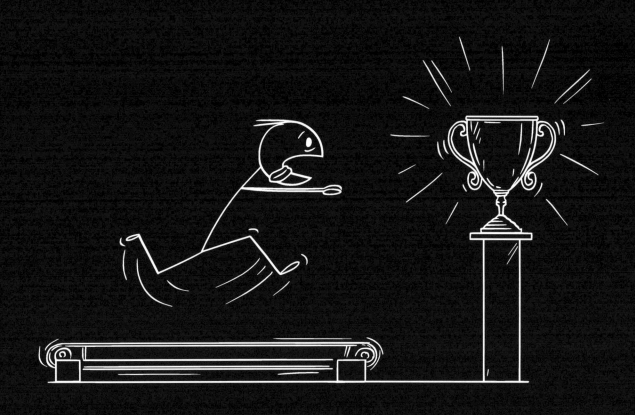

Forced Achievement vs. Inevitable Achievement

"After putting the right systems
and tools in place...
Irregardless of inconsistencies in
my mindset
Remain consistent in my actions
The BIRTH of my dreams is not
only possible, it becomes
inevitable"

- Tessa Aranda

IT WAS A HOT, muggy morning, and my body was screaming at me as I laced up my shoes and looked at my running schedule. 'Run 3 miles today,' it said. 'Are you kidding me?' I thought to myself. Running a half marathon seemed like a far-off wish, something honestly terrifying to have to do. But I just showed up, turning on my GPS map and my music, and I left.

I ran at a slow and steady pace, sometimes speeding up with the downslope or a fun song, sometimes doing sprints if that's what my app asked me to do. In the beginning, getting to the point where I could run the race felt impossible. But every day, I showed up, and I ran a little bit farther.

Then one day, a little past halfway through my training, something changed. I ran 8 miles for the first time, and as I finished, I had this profound moment of knowing that running and completing the 13.1 mile race was inevitable. It was as if I already ran the race. I was becoming a marathoner.

After I hit that tipping point, my mind was totally free. It wasn't about having to dig in to run farther than I ever had; I actually knew that I could run anything that was on my half marathon training schedule. And every day, as I finished up mile one, I settled into my old familiar flow. I was no longer running to try to do something anymore. I had become a runner.

It's the same with motherhood. You can reach leverage points and stop forcing success in so many areas of your life. Maybe it's the rhythm of lighthearted conversation you've developed with your budding teenager, or the zones in your home that you can easily maintain that bring a sense of peace and order. Once you hit that tipping point, where you know that you can do it, the ball starts rolling itself. You become a mom who can handle anything that comes her way.

Setting goals that make you a better mother is a great way to shift your focus from striving for success to creating momentum and flow in your life. The key is to set realistic, achievable goals that align with your values and priorities as a mother, to stick with them, and to hold out hope that you will not have to maintain those new ways of being on sheer willpower forever.

Strength of will is an incredible character trait that I value and always desire. But I know myself well enough that instead of relying on that willpower in most areas of my life, I create and follow systems that develop the mental, emotional and physical 'muscle memory' that will get me to the tipping point, and allow inevitable success. There is infinite joy and ease in inevitability. I'll trade that in for force any day.

For example, you might set a goal to spend more quality time with your children, whether that means planning a weekly family outing or dedicating a certain amount of time each day to play with your kids. Or, you might set a goal to prioritize self-care, such as getting more sleep, exercising regularly, or making time for hobbies and activities that bring you joy.

The important thing is to start small and build momentum over time. This was the key to my 'buy-in' for a half marathon. Because all I had to do was install an app, that today, I woke up, and ran the one mile it told me. Rather than obsessing about the lofty-far off goal, focus on small, manageable changes that you can incorporate daily. As you begin to make progress towards your goals, you'll start to feel a sense of momentum and flow in your life. You start to become 'an early riser' after a consistent 2 weeks of setting your alarm, you start to become a more lighthearted mother as you practice laughing intentionally throughout your day.

Once you've been consistent with your new habits for a while, you may reach a tipping point where you start to feel a sense of inevitability about your success. This is when your habits become second nature, and you no longer have to force yourself to make time for self-care or spend quality time with your children. It becomes a natural part of your routine, and you feel more in control of your life and your motherhood journey.

To help reach this tipping point, it can be helpful to track your progress and celebrate your successes along the way. This can help you stay motivated and focused on your goals, even when the going gets tough. Apps are my favorite, and many people love habit trackers in print out form (slap in on the fridge or next to your bed!). Remember, it's okay to have setbacks and slip-ups along the way. What's important is that you keep moving forward and stay committed to your goals, even when progress is slow.

This concept of inevitable success due to consistency and hitting a tipping point is based on the idea that success can become inevitable if you consistently take action towards your goal and eventually hit a point where momentum takes over. If you love this idea and want to saturate yourself in the belief of inevitable success several thought leaders explore these concepts in different contexts, including Malcolm Gladwell in his book "The Tipping Point," James Clear in his book "Atomic Habits," and Steven Pressfield in his book "The War of Art".

What big fun goal would you set if you knew success was inevitable? What daily action systems would you need to put in place for that goal? Start thinking of new systems that may move you toward your big goal to begin integrating into your life in the right season.

LEVERAGE POINT
(WHEN SUCCESS BECOMES INEVITABLE)

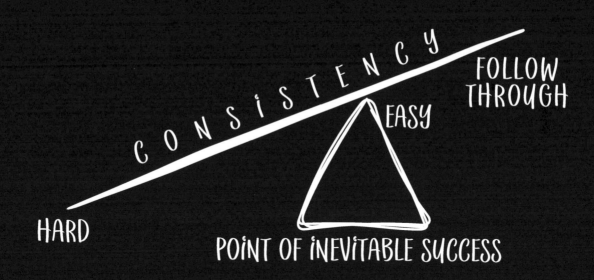

9. CELEBRA
NOT PER

TE PROCESS

FECTION

Yay! Process!

LET'S TALK ABOUT THE world's obsession with 'Progress over Perfection' - it's everywhere! But let's be real, it's not as easy as it sounds, especially for us women and mamas. We're wired to strive for perfection and completion, and progress can feel like a far-off dream. So, we need to shift our mindset and celebrate the process, not just the end result. It's in the process that we grow, learn, and ultimately create something extraordinary. When we only focus on completion and perfection, we miss out on the joy and fulfillment that comes with the journey.

But the process can be messy. Super messy, imperfect, flawed. We laid the foundation with daily imperfect action, flailing, learning to own and befriend our shadow, all of this in an effort to embrace and love the process of the mess. Enduring the mess while still resisting it, rather than embracing it, keeps us reliant on our traditional aim for progress and perfection which ultimately robs us from experiencing the joy and ease that come with letting go of that resistance. If we can't learn to loosen our grip on our conditioned resistance to imperfection, we won't ever fully experience presence and joy in the process.

So, how do we fix this? It's simple: focus on the process, not just the end result. The journey is just as important as the destination. When we celebrate each step along the way and who we are becoming, we open ourselves up to more joy, flow, and ease. However, when we focus only on progress, we may fall back into old patterns of judging ourselves harshly for not progressing enough, which can lead to shame and self-doubt. By celebrating the process, we can see the beauty in the messy middle, the mistakes and the missteps, and learn from them with a broader perspective.

Celebrating the little wins along the way is essential to begin putting process over perfection. If you're working on a big project, celebrate the fact that you made progress by completing a portion of the project, even if it's not yet finished. Acknowledge the effort and time you put into it, and feel proud of yourself for taking action towards your goal.

I love acknowledging the process and all the mess by celebrating at the end of the day with a Ta-Da list. How many times do you look back on your week like– 'What did I even do this week? I know I was busy- but I don't feel fulfilled or complete.' Often, being able to experience fulfillment comes through acknowledgement, not necessarily progress. It's about being kind to yourself, recognizing that progress and accomplishment are not always linear, and finding joy and satisfaction in the journey. Celebrating that growth, knowledge, and becoming are gained along the way, and not just at the moment of completion.

In the parable of a Quantity vs. Quality study[4] participants were divided into two groups: one group was instructed to create a single, perfect ceramic pot, while the other group was asked to create as many pots as possible within a set time limit. Interestingly, the group that was focused on quantity ended up producing not only more pots, but also better quality ones.

This story illustrates an important lesson that can be applied to many areas of life, including motherhood: sometimes, the pursuit of perfection can actually hold us back from achieving our goals. When we are too focused on getting things 'right,' we can become paralyzed by fear of failure and end up doing nothing at all.

On the other hand, when we give ourselves permission to make mistakes and focus on quantity over quality, we can actually achieve more and even surprise ourselves with the quality of our work. This approach can help us get things done and feel a greater sense of accomplishment, which can be incredibly empowering.

So as a mom, try embracing imperfection and focusing on simply getting things done, rather than obsessing over every detail. Remember, sometimes the pursuit of perfection can actually hold us back, while embracing imperfection can lead to greater success and fulfillment.

When it comes to feeding your kids, celebrating the process can mean trying out new recipes, involving them in meal planning and preparation, and making mealtime a fun and educational experience. By focusing on the process, you can feel more joy and less stress, and your kids are more likely to develop healthy habits over time.

One example of celebrating the process could be acknowledging the effort and dedication you put into a task, even if the end result isn't perfect or fully completed. If you set a goal to exercise every day but miss a few days due to unexpected events, celebrate the fact that you made an effort to exercise on most days and recognize the obstacles that got in the way. Take note of what worked and what didn't work, and adjust your approach to be more effective in the future.

The key is to focus on the journey, rather than the destination. Whether it's in your career, your relationships, or your personal pursuits, take pride in the steps you're taking each day to improve and grow. Let me be obnoxious and say it one more time: True joy and fulfillment come from embracing the process, not just the end result. From the mama who lets my kids smear paint in their hair if that's what it takes for expression and joy, I give you permission to let loose. Let's get messy y'all.

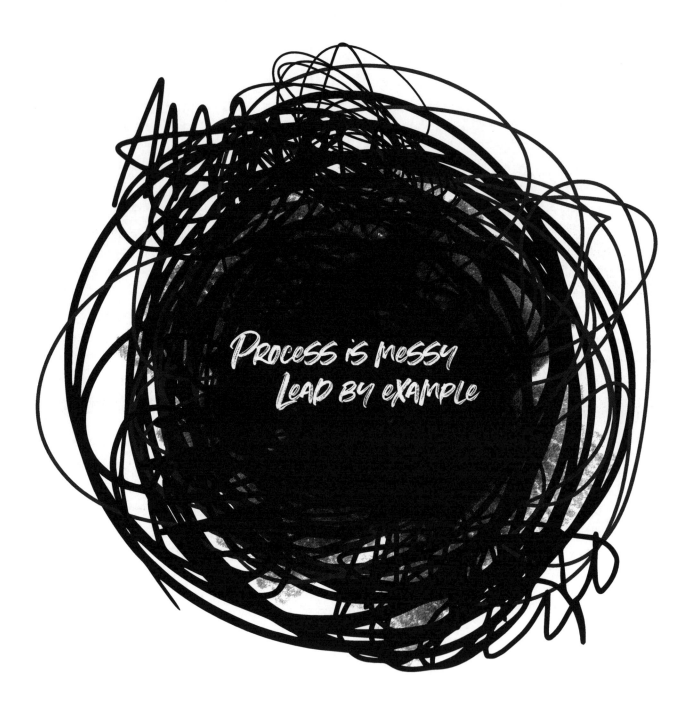

Healing Our Perception Of Cycles And Time

LET'S TALK ABOUT CYCLES, rhythms, and time - and how we can shift our perception of them to unlock our power to create more time in our lives. Yes, you heard me right - you have the power to create more time!

First of all, let's recognize that time is cyclical. It's not a straight line from point A to point B. Think about a clock - it's round for a reason. When we 'lose' an hour and we are thinking linearly, we are in a desperate race to completion before we reach the end of our rope. Our rope keeps getting cut shorter and shorter (a lot of times while feeling that we have no control). Instead, if we see the 360 degree view of time that feeds continually back into itself, we have a constant renewal of 24 hours at our disposal. When it comes to a linear perception of time, it's easy to get caught up focusing on what we've lost or where we fell short. But if we can shift our focus to viewing time as an infinite vortex, never ending and unrestrictive, our concept of what is possible opens up and becomes limitless. The illustration on the next page may help to check in with how you have been perceiving time, and what other possibilities exist.

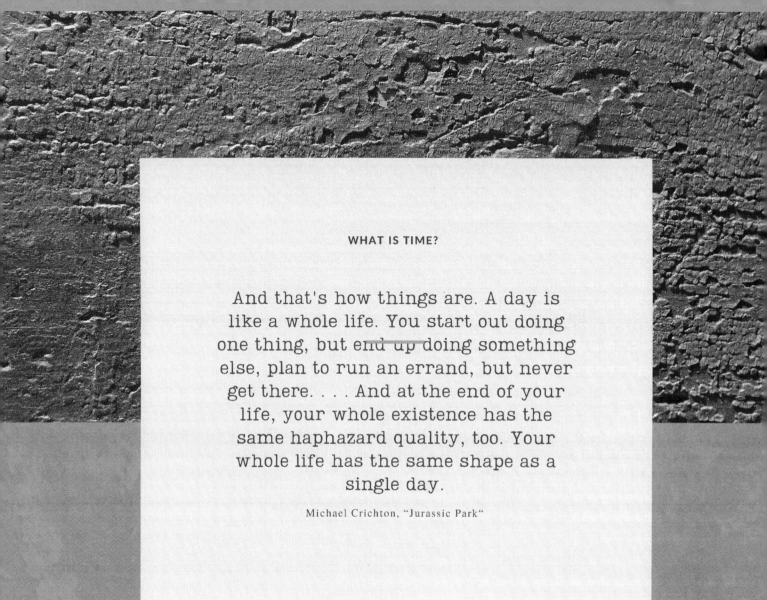

WHAT IS TIME?

And that's how things are. A day is
like a whole life. You start out doing
one thing, but ~~end up~~ doing something
else, plan to run an errand, but never
get there. . . . And at the end of your
life, your whole existence has the
same haphazard quality, too. Your
whole life has the same shape as a
single day.

Michael Crichton, "Jurassic Park"

As moms, we often feel like time is a scarce resource that we are constantly competing to manage. However, by shifting our perspective and seeing time as a renewable resource that moves in cycles, we can experience more joy and ease in even the most mundane tasks like cleaning the kitchen.

The vortex is a state of being where we can slow down time and enter a state of hyper-focus, where distractions and anxieties around time disappear. By learning to be present in the moment, we can tap into this flow state and experience a sense of control over time. This allows us to feel more in control of our lives and experience more joy and ease in our daily activities.

When cleaning the kitchen, for example, we can use the vortex to slow down time and focus on the task at hand. Rather than feeling rushed or overwhelmed, we can enter a flow state where we enjoy the process of cleaning and feel a sense of accomplishment as we complete the task. This experience of the vortex can be applied to any task, no matter how mundane, and can help us experience more joy and ease in our daily lives.

As we practice entering the vortex, we come to realize that what we do with our time is a choice, and we are not victims of time. This realization can be liberating and empowering, allowing us to feel more in control of our lives and experience more joy and ease in our daily activities. So, next time you're cleaning the kitchen, try entering the vortex and see how it can transform the experience for you.

That might have gotten a little woo woo for you but spend some time with it, it might surprise you. Aside from all that, we all have certain habits that dictate the way we interact with time. We have good habits, bad habits, and everything in between. We also have seasons of new beginnings, growth, and abundance, and seasons of stillness, emptiness, and letting go. These patterns exist not just in our lives, but in the world around us - from generational cycles to menstrual cycles to motherhood cycles.

Here's the thing, though - we have the power to create the life of joy and accomplishment that we desire, no matter what season or cycle we're in. It all comes down to awareness and acceptance. When we're unconscious of or resistant to our cyclical patterns, we're at the mercy of them. But when we discover and embrace them, we can create with ease.

For example, let's say you're feeling stuck in a cycle of overwhelm and stress. Instead of fighting against it, try to embrace it as a season of stillness and rest. Allow yourself to slow down, take a break, and recharge. When you're ready, you can begin to take small steps forward and gradually build momentum.

Or maybe you're in a season of new beginnings, and you're ready to take on a new project or pursue a new goal. Rather than getting caught up in the end result, focus on the process and enjoy the journey. Celebrate the small wins along the way, and trust that the end result will come in due time.

Remember, our cyclical patterns are not a sign of failure or falling short. They are a natural part of life, and when we learn to work with them, we can unlock our true power and potential. So embrace your cycles, embrace your rhythms, and create the life you deserve! Time is on your side my friend.

Time Perception

WE ALWAYS HAVE A CHOICE

Linear: Limited

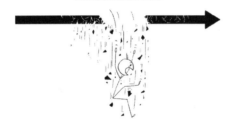

**Vortex: No End
Infinite**

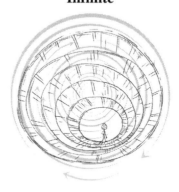

**Cyclical:
Renewable 24 hours**

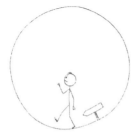

WEAKNESS IS A GIFT THAT ALLOWS US TO CREATE PROCESSES

LET'S FLIP THE SCRIPT on weakness and turn it into a powerful tool for creating unstoppable processes. See, I've been chasing physical goals for as long as I can remember. Building strength, shedding pounds - you know the drill. And I quickly learned that the only way to achieve lasting change is through consistency. As someone who has loved starting things but struggled with consistency my whole life, that's where the struggle came in. Trying to overcome our weaknesses on sheer willpower is a losing battle. So what's the solution? Processes.

Back in 'Forced Success vs Inevitable Success,' I talked about the power of systems that make success inevitable. The key is finding the right processes that work for us and implementing them quickly. No wasting time with trial and error. But how do we do that without burning out and losing faith in ourselves?

Here's where weakness comes in. It's not something to be ashamed of or hide from - it's the key to unlocking our potential. Think of it as a map of your life. By understanding our weaknesses and strengths, we can map out the processes that will support us on our journey.

Processes are like the step-by-step guide to achieving a specific goal or task, while a system is the big picture of all those processes working together in harmony. To build your own system, you need to first understand your own habits and cycles, and then love and accept them. Embrace your winter slump and use it as an opportunity to study your energy patterns. That way, when your productive, energetic beast mode kicks in, you're ready to maximize that momentum.

But here's the catch - before you can create processes that will work for you, you need to acknowledge and surrender to your own weaknesses. Once you're aware of your own energy, ability, and desires, you can stop forcing yourself into behaviors that don't fit and start seeking out new possibilities. It's a practice that requires patience and self-compassion, but the payoff is huge. With the right processes in place, you'll be unstoppable.

THE KINTSUGI SELF

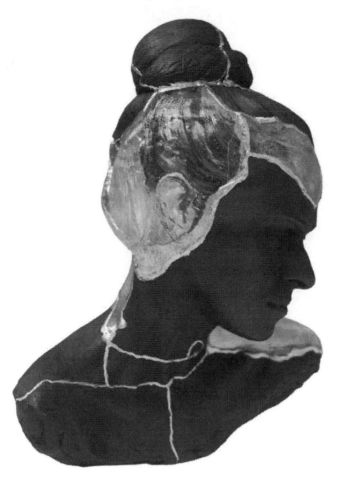

HAVE YOU EVER HEARD of kintsugi? It's a mesmerizing art form that celebrates the beauty of imperfection. But here's the kicker - the stunning results of kintsugi would never have come to be if the pottery wasn't first shattered into pieces. That's right, the beauty of kintsugi lies in its brokenness.

You see, when a piece of pottery breaks, it's often considered useless and thrown away. But in the art of kintsugi, those broken pieces are carefully and lovingly put back together using a special lacquer mixed with gold, silver, or platinum. The resulting piece is not only restored, but it's also transformed into something uniquely beautiful.

And that's the thing about kintsugi - the beauty lies not only in the finished product but also in the process of putting it back together. The creator has the freedom to exercise their creativity in a way that embraces the imperfections and creates something truly one-of-a-kind. And for the viewer, the shattered and restored art piece serves as a reminder that brokenness can be transformed into something stunning and that imperfections can be celebrated.

Just as the completed kintsugi pottery is transformed into something even more beautiful because of its brokenness, a mother's weaknesses can ultimately make her a stronger and more resilient parent. By embracing her weaknesses and using them to develop processes and strategies that work for her family, she can become a more effective and compassionate mother, with a gorgeous life adorned in gold.

When I decided to train for my first half marathon, I knew I had a weakness of getting excited about something, then quickly getting bored and quitting. So, to ensure I didn't give up on this goal, I decided to put processes in place to make sure I stayed motivated and consistent.

First, I signed up for the race with two friends who were also training. We would Marco Polo each other every day to share our progress and keep each other accountable. This helped me stay committed to the goal even on days when I didn't feel like running.

Second, I relied on an app that told me exactly how far and how to run every day. I didn't have to make any decisions, or rely on my own sense of motivation or daily desire to effect what would happen that day. I just did what It said to do and trusted that if i followed the plan, I would be prepared for the race. I gave myself grace and ran super slow some days (I'm talkin 15 min miles that my husband jokes looked like fast walking), and even let myself pause my app and rest to walk for 10 minutes on the occasional difficult 10 mile run. I allowed the system I put in place to be for me, allowing grace and surrender, while still sticking to it.

Third, I signed up for shorter races in the months leading up to the half marathon. This allowed me to leverage accountability to 'someone else' (in this case the actual race I had committed to) and celebrate who I was becoming through the process. The victories that I celebrated along the way were not just my progress in pace or distance, but who I was becoming in the process of training. I was making my weakest parts strong. And I'm not just talking about my legs! I was becoming consistent. I was becoming a person who made promises and commitments to myself, and I kept them. And how I was with myself I started being everywhere. I was more reliable and committed to others as well. The process was what was changing me, not the race. I woke up every day feeling different, and that sense of becoming, ironically, helped me stay motivated and focused on the end goal.

Finally, I habit stacked my running time as my 'me' time away from my kids. I would listen to podcasts, catch up with friends, and even write marketing posts with voice to text while I ran. This made my running time my favorite part of the day, and it helped me stay consistent with my training.

By putting these processes in place, I was able to overcome my weakness of quitting and complete my first half marathon. And even more than that, I developed a love for running and a habit of consistent exercise that I still maintain to this day. Every process I put in place in my life builds ease and flow into my life while building character where I before felt weak. Screw it- I know I sound like a broken record, loving our mediocrity, unlocks everything!

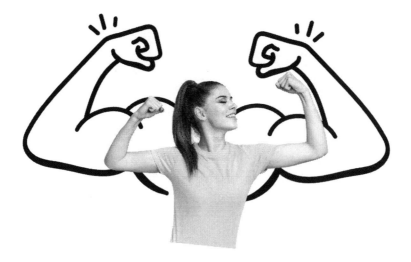

Stop Being a Machine and Start Building Them

IT'S THE MOMENT WE'VE been waiting for! You know what they say, delegation is key to creating more ease and flow in your life and family. The first step is to stop being okay with being a machine. Recognize that you've taken on too much unnecessarily and that there are systems and processes that you can build today, which can take off up to 80% of your workload in various areas of your life. You were never meant to be a machine, you were meant to build them!

There are millions of ways you can delegate your work as a mom and create machines or systems that work for you and your family. The actual machines I have built that are working for me and my family, don't actually matter for you. (Although you can find a list of my favorites on www.mediocremommagic.com under 'freebies'— the list includes the meal planner I had a vision of and changed my life). So, what will make a difference and help you build the absolute best machines in your life for more ease and contentment? Looking at why they are not in place now.

Here are the various reasons you may not have machines and you are stuck burning your candle at both ends trying to be the machine running everything in everyone's life:

You aren't seeing where they can be put in place.

You don't know which machine to use.

It feels exhausting and like a lot of work to put a new machine in place.

The machine relies on other people (either to create it or keep it running).

The very nature of our roles as house and mother is to teach and to impart our knowledge and wisdom. Mothers simply do much more than they need to, and in doing so deprive the home of integration, progress, and efficiency, as well as depriving the children of the opportunities to grow and strengthen their skills in cooperation, collaboration, following a system, and eventually building systems themselves that can be taught and followed.

Now, you may be reading this and saying, 'Oh, my kids know their responsibilities, and they, for sure, help out.' But obeying an assignment is very different from obeying the steps of a well-proven system and learning the skills to develop, initiate, and train others on their own systems that save them time and energy.

Our work as mothers is and has always been building the machines to keep our world running. To build them better (more efficiently), to teach their usage, and to create progress, flow, and ease in our homes. If we are feeling overloaded, under-appreciated, creatively dead inside, or just downright overwhelmed, it would likely do us much good to notice if we are in practice of being a machine or creating them.

Now, once we recognize we are doing much too much in any one area or any task, we can tap into possibilities and ask these key questions shown on the next page to decide what machine needs to be built. Before we dive into those, though, we must first address the elephant in the room. I am promising here that building a machine will create up to 80% less work for you, yes. And, the tinkering and testing, and trial period, and integration of the machine into your family's processes will definitely take more effort. It may feel at first that it is just less work to continue doing something the old way or all by yourself when you see all the effort that it takes to put it in place. You've probably attempted the creation of machines many times before and given up because of this very fact.

The question you must ask yourself is, 'Am I willing to put the work in now, to sit back and do 80% less work forever in this area?' Forever. Those people that developed the innovations that led to the automatic washing machine, freed women up to have more choice as to what to do with their time. Just as the washboard scrubbin' women before us earned back so much more physical time by building machines and delegating tasks, you can free up your physical and emotional energy and focus on the things that truly matter to you by doing the same. Plus, you can teach your children important life skills and instill a sense of teamwork and collaboration in your family.

So if you're feeling overwhelmed, it's time to start building those machines! Ask yourself the key questions on the next page, and use the answers to guide you in creating systems that will work for you and your family. It may take some effort and trial and error, but the payoff of having more ease and flow in your life is well worth it.

Questions For Your Machine

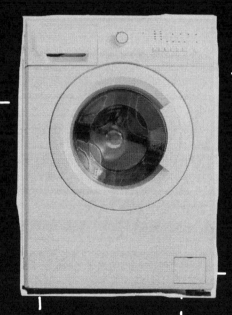

Will it take 80% of the task off my plate?

Which "model" is right for me & my family?

Is there a system for training others in how to use it?

How are others using it to do less and get more done?

If applicable: How do you clean it?

10. FIND
THE WORLD

THE MAGIC

IS FULL OF IT

Everyone Is A Creative Genius

HUMANS ARE CREATIVE. CREATIVITY is not a skill, or a talent some select few are born with. Creativity is the magic ability of seeing possibilities. 'Artists' or 'Creative Professionals' are humans that are used to processing ideas in a certain way. They don't have more ideas, they are just used to capturing them, sorting through, then making something that endures. (Which is basically the process of learning motherhood, right?) Most ideas aren't good. Every human has tons of bad ideas. But those we call creative are simply the people who have habits and processes to record and review those ideas later, then take massive action and create 'Big Fun' in their lives by following through. In taking imperfect action on those discovered 'worthwhile ideas' they become known as creatives. Basically, they take more shots, so they score more p oints.

Inspiration does not happen inside a vacuum. Creation is born by spending time in introspection, which then leads to progress, and completion. Creating the mediocre magical you that feels more fulfilled, joyful and at ease requires this type of creativity. Reflection allows you to become more 'Extra' in your ordinary ness.

I'm curious, do you go back to your habits and review? Or even back to those sweet and precious moments that we, maybe, rushed through and regret missing in the moment? Last time it was a rainy day did you grumble at the idea of having to be stuck indoors all day? Or did you start to see more possibilities? If you just move on, living in those moments, without reviewing what else could have been (not what should have been!), but what could have been- you lose the opportunity to find the magic, find your creative processing skills, and become the createtress of your life.

People want to know how I write so often. Have such profound lessons and metaphors and share hope through the imperfection of my life. It is not something I can teach my clients to do. Sure, there are tools, writing strategies, keys like writing as if you are speaking to a friend, but, it is through the practice and decision of writing every day that the marketer learns the skill of seeing the lessons all around them every day that can be transformed and transmitted in a powerful way to their audience.

The problem is not that you are not inspired, the problem is that most moms are so busy they don't realize when inspiration is happening. They have an idea in their minds of what being a 'creative mom' or a 'present mom' looks like, and those ideas are not necessarily true. Inspiration, ideas, creativity is much more common than we realize. We all are much more likely to mistake 'inspiration' for just our thoughts and to not burrow down into the rabbit hole of magic that it presents. Inspiration, revelation, creation, magic, involves a lot more work, and not just sitting there getting information. You must demand inspiration. You know how they say if it's a priority but you don't put it on your calendar it won't happen? The same goes for inspiration. Make it a priority to recognize, capture, voice memo, take note, share with a friend. Make listening to your genius (the Roman one) part of your daily flow.

Have you ever heard 'it's hard for God to steer a parked car'? Many of us, myself included, will wait for inspiration, and that's not how it comes. I dread bedtime, almost every night. And, I also crave a deeper connection with my children. Sending them off to bed then spending 'me time' sitting on the couch pondering ideas of how to connect to them more deeply rarely works for me. It's like staring at a blank canvas.

Instead, when I go lay down for a quick snuggle chat, it's like laying down a first layer of paint. I have something to respond to. Something that moves and is varied and is interesting. Every word from their mouth inspires deeper connection, and gives me clues and inner pings of revelation on what that child needs. You cannot wait to get your brush dirty until after the magic comes. It's waiting for you to get dirty and get to work.

Inspiration

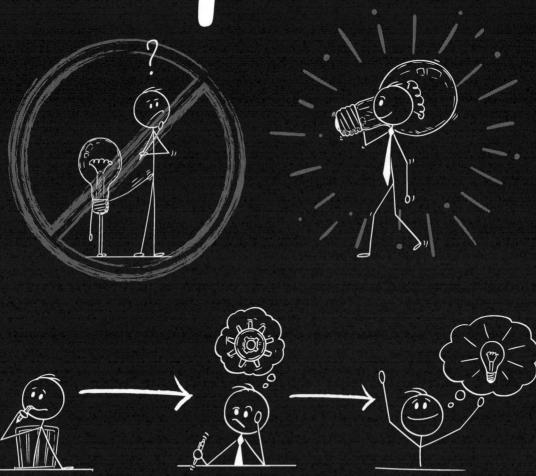

EXPANDERS

LET'S EXPLORE BEING EXPANDED by the law of the mirror. Remember that your brain can't decipher subconsciously if what you are seeing is your life or someone else? Have you ever heard of the saying, 'You are the sum of the 5 people you spend the most time with'? This is the most exciting thing! You can hack your creative genius by using this law of the mirror. You can become a more expanded version of yourself by seeing more often who you want to become.

Who do you know that you see as wildly creative, fun, carefree, or present in their life, their work, or with their children? Make a list of the things you have seen her do that were magical to you. They are likely ordinary moments. And they may have even been moments that you found yourself comparing. When we feel jealousy or comparison it is a sign or gift to us that our subconscious knows that all those same things are available to us, now. It supports us when we know that she is both powerful in her joy, and that she can be that joyful, flowing mother even with her flaws and challenges. These are the diamond expanders in our lives. Because it becomes more possible for us. She does these things in spite of her imperfections- not because she doesn't have any.

Make a list of those moments with the intention of being inspired and expanded. This list is a key not to doing but to becoming. Not doing what she does but seeing how she sees. Being in each moment, more of who you want to be. You do not have to do what she does, but see how she sees. See possibility, opportunity, and growth in each moment with yourself and your kids. Next time you have a moment with your children you know you are dragging your feet, dreading, or hoping you can just get through alive, check in and ask, "What Would She See?"

Not what she would do, but what possibilities would she see? This is where the magic lives, you just have to find it.

THE MAGIC OF EXPANSION

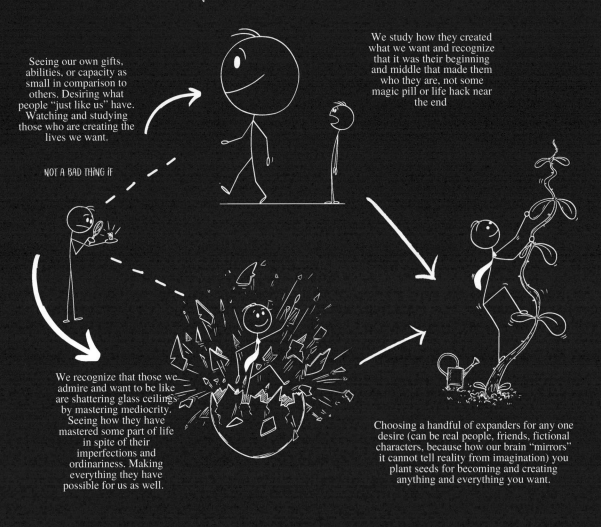

Seeing our own gifts, abilities, or capacity as small in comparison to others. Desiring what people "just like us" have. Watching and studying those who are creating the lives we want.

NOT A BAD THING IF

We study how they created what we want and recognize that it was their beginning and middle that made them who they are, not some magic pill or life hack near the end

We recognize that those we admire and want to be like are shattering glass ceilings by mastering mediocrity. Seeing how they have mastered some part of life in spite of their imperfections and ordinariness. Making everything they have possible for us as well.

Choosing a handful of expanders for any one desire (can be real people, friends, fictional characters, because how our brain "mirrors" it cannot tell reality from imagination) you plant seeds for becoming and creating anything and everything you want.

~~Appreciation~~ Discovery

OH MAKE SURE YOU appreciate it,' is probably the worst and most annoying advice that moms ever get. When we are told we simply must appreciate our current state of affairs when we are struggling, we only feel more shame, more frustration, confusion, and like we are not enough. We feel hopeless to find any true path to ease, joy, contentment. In fact, we may even begin to believe that ease, joy, and contentment do not exist for mothers. Appreciation, for most moms, is too big of a leap in belief. We need that bridge of belief or of evidence to get us there. The biggest flaw with this destructive advice for mothers is that appreciation is a decision, not a destination.

An easier, much more readily available decision for moms that leads to the result of appreciation, joy, ease, flow, all the yummy things... is the decision to Discover. To choose to be in the value of discovery daily. Discovery is a magical, potent decision to observe and find and see what already is. To see what we maybe were not seeing before. To seek and to find daily.

I love abstract painting...

Just as I put paint to canvas, releasing expectations of what I will create and allow what is already there to be discovered, delighted in and shared, we as moms can put paint to the canvas of our lives and enjoy the happy accidents. We can delight in the varying light and dark, the unexpected drips and color combinations that lend beauty and cohesiveness in a way that we could never have planned. We can release the pressure to create the Magic, and bask in the reassurance that when we take imperfect action daily, with eyes of discovery, we can learn to see, and experience delight daily.

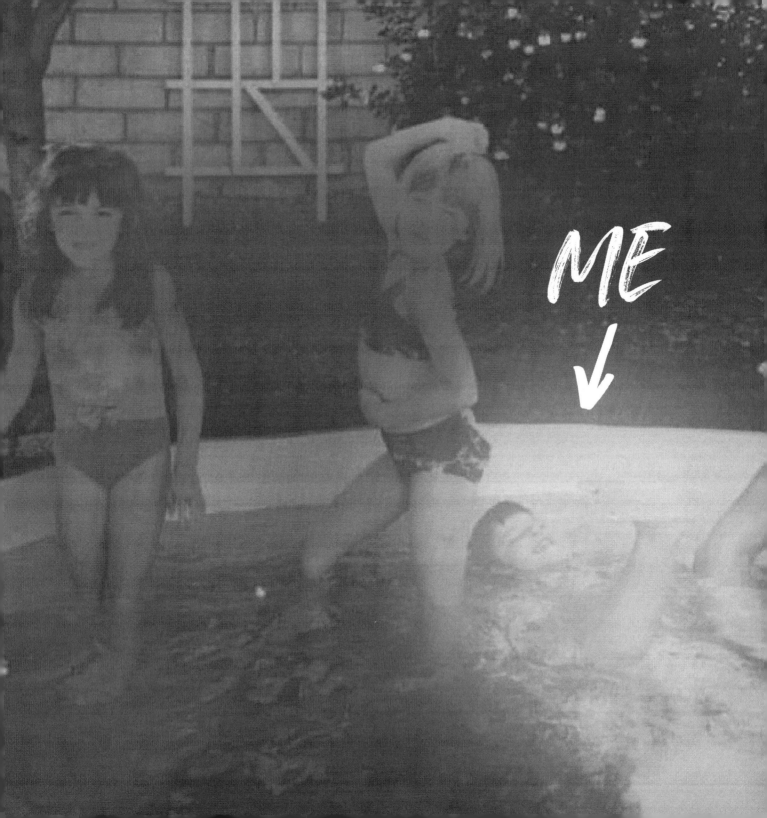

ME
↓

Choose Delight

I HAVE A FRIEND, Suzy that often would say to me how delightful it was to watch her sweet little Abigail as she grew. She would tell me a story and I could feel the warmth and expansion and joy that came in the simple observation of her child. This was something, I thought, I had never experienced before. The recognizing and recollecting of a delightful moment. That word changed everything for me.

But then I realized something - delight could be mine too! I began to ask myself, "how can I delight in my children?" and started to pay attention to the simple moments of their being. Their questions, their expressions, even the things that used to irritate me became opportunities for me to experience delight.

Maybe 'delight' isn't the value word that resonates with you, but the key is to find a value word that shifts your perspective and helps you to be intentional and awake in the present moment. Whether it's 'discovery' or 'flow,' the magic lies in seeing and being, not in more doing and striving. As you explore, I want to illustrate your powerful ability to receive the exact words that are right for you.

Affirmations vs Afformations

WHY ARE SO MANY women reclaiming their mediocrity and joining us in the Mediocre Moms Club? I believe it's because we're tired of feeling like we're not enough, like we have to be perfect all the time. Words like 'mediocre' and 'imperfect' have been used to tear us down, but we're taking back the power and using them to build ourselves up. And it's not just about us as individuals. It's about our lives and our circumstances.

A 'mediocre life' doesn't have to be a bad thing. In fact, it can be a beautiful thing, full of simplicity and magic in the little moments. When we allow ourselves to be still and surrender, we open ourselves up to more joy, ease, and flow in our day-to-day lives. It's time to embrace the magic of mediocrity and seek deeper fulfillment in our lives. And the best part? It's available to every mom, everywhere. Words hold immense power, and as we navigate through life, we have the choice to shape our experiences through the words we choose to use. This is where the concept of diction comes into play, and it emphasizes the power of choice. We have the power to make our words mean whatever we want them to mean, even transforming a word like "mediocre" to symbolize alignment, growth, and letting go of perfectionism. Let's shake off the shackles of "shoulds" and trust our intuition, because deep down, we all have the answers we need within ourselves.

How, then, do we harness the power of our intuition and transform our mediocrity into something empowering? A daily restorative practice and affirmations can be a great place to start, but you know how I feel about affirmations (not my fave, y'all! Here's why—-) While affirmations have their place, if we are telling our subconscious, our spirit, our minds that we are enough, we are not leaving room to receive what we truly are. We are force feeding and stuffing our heads so full, we miss the magic. We need to move beyond simply repeating "I am enough" and instead ask ourselves what it truly means to be enough. Defining our values and how they relate to feeling "enough" is a vital step in our journey of self-discovery. Instead, healing questions can help us explore our values and visualize what it truly means to embody them. The problem is traditional affirmations can fall short if our subconscious is not aligned with them. This is where afformations come in - they are questions we ask ourselves that engage our brains in formulating solutions and affirmations specific to us. These questions serve as a healing tool to guide, comfort, and affirm us by listening to the innate responses from our subconscious mind. This technique can help us tap into the wisdom that our spirit possesses, even when we consciously feel discomfort or confusion. In essence, afformations help us to access our own inner wisdom and guidance, allowing us to find the answers that we need to live our best lives. They can be a powerful tool for self-discovery, healing, and growth. And finding the magic (remember...the world is full of it)!

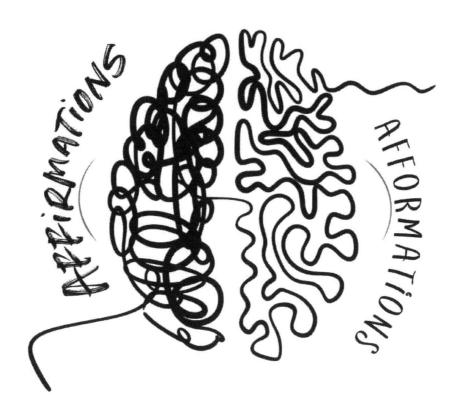

TESSA'S AFFORMATIONS FOR MEDIOCRE MAMAS

AFFORMATIONS FOR...

When you are feeling/believing that you are not doing or being enough.

- What if this is exactly what the world/my family/my home/myself needs me to show up as right now?

- What if there is no such thing as enough, what would I do differently?

- Why do I feel fulfilled?

- Why am I exactly where I need to be?

- In what ways am I so present in this moment?

- How can I let go of doing, and just be?

- What one thing does my higher power (God) want me to focus on right now?

- How am I experiencing my values and genius in what I'm choosing?

- How can I choose into my values?

When you feel like you are too much.

- How am I exactly what this world/family/group/space needs right now?

- How is the space supporting my full expression?

- What expression am I allowing myself to fully experience in this moment?

- How am I creating movement for others?

- How am I creating some fun discomfort for others?

- How am I creating light and expansion for others?

- What are others learning from me in my 'extra'-ness?

When your life does not feel like enough

- Why is the ordinary so delightful to me today?

- How am I so able to be present to what brings me joy?

- What is expanding in my life?

- What is possible for me today?

- How is today growing me?

- Why do I feel so fulfilled?

- How is the void supporting my future creation?

- Why is joy and ease abundant in my life?

- How am I so good at letting go and being content where I am?

When your life feels like too much.
- Why is peace so abundant in my life?

- How am I so good at learning from my circumstances?

- Why is my growth so easy right now?

- Why is my weakness such a gift?

- Why am I so good at asking for the support I need?

- Why is my life so abundant with opportunity?

- How is my life a gift of growth?

When you feel Creatively dead inside.
- Why (or how) am I inspired today?

- Why is the world around me so inspiring?

- How do I feel connected today?

- What ideas can I capture today?

- What is there for me to discover in this moment?

- Why is my body and mind so supportive of creation?

When you are triggered.

- Why am I learning and healing so much right now?

- Why is this so expansive?

- How am I able to be so present with myself in this moment?

- How is it so easy to surrender and receive what I need?

- Why are my values so supportive to me in this moment?

All the time...

- What if there's nothing wrong here?

- What if everything is going right here?

- What if I choose ease in this moment?

So What Now, Lady?

ALRIGHT, MY DEAR MEDIOCRE Moms, it's time for our grand finale! As we come to the end of this book, I want you to take a deep breath and congratulate yourself. You've come a long way, and you should be gosh dern proud of yourself!

But let me tell you, the journey is far from over. Motherhood is a never-ending adventure that requires constant learning, growth, and support. That's why I want to invite you to keep using this book as your reference toolkit/guide to motherhood. Remember the book is laid out to facilitate a new way of thinking, a new way of being, and finally, a new way of doing.

As you come back to sections you need again and again, just know, you never have to do this alone. You've got a whole community of Mediocre Moms standing right beside you, cheering you on every step of the way. So, share this book with your friends, keep the conversation alive, and join us at Mediocremomsclub.com to join the actual club.

And that's not all. I invite you to delve deeper into each chapter every single week on the podcast, Mediocre Moms Club. We'll explore these tools even further, share our wins, our struggles, and our moments of magic.

Now, let's not forget the magic that comes when you use these tools. Understanding why mediocrity is magical, being extra at being ordinary, restoration vs. rest, momming 'who you are', doing vs. being, rear-view visioning with values in mind, being willing to have fun getting uncomfortable, creating big fun, celebrating process over perfection, and always finding the magic.

My dear Mediocre Moms, you've got this. You are powerful, strong, and capable of creating the life you want for yourself and your family. So, keep using these tools, keep growing, and keep shining. I believe in you!

Acknowledgements

I want to send so much love and gratitude to all the current, future, and forever masters of the magically mediocre– the moms. Especially those dear friends who held my hand through this grueling process and were my biggest cheerleaders along the way Charla, Arielle, Gina, Meghan, Andrea, Amy, Emily, Rebekah, Kerry, and Maci. Without your input and enthusiasm none of this would have been possible. To my editors who came in clutch at the last minute in droves: Lynda, Silke, Marissa, and Charla, my relentlessly loving critic & the gracious Yael. Arielle for being my sounding board from conception, Charla for being my best and most powerful critical eye, encourager, and best friend, and Meghan for being as excited about this book as I hope all moms will be. This book would not have been possible without the three of you. To my five sweet children who gave me so much grace in my mediocrity throughout the birth of this book.

To Beth and Jen for changing my brain and my mothering forever. To all of my clients and team members over the last decade for always seeing my strength, trusting my guidance, and being willing to get Funcomfortable to birth a more creative, expansive life and business. You are my biggest inspiration. And always, to my biggest supporter and forever lover, Bub. Thank you for always seeing the magic in my hair brained dreaming. For holding my hand when I am broken and encouraging me to see my greatness and become better. I love doing life with you.

BIBLIOGRAPHY

1. Barker, Kirsten.. "Quantity Breeds Quality." BoFa Institute for the Foundations of Animal Behavior, Cornell University, 22 June 2006, https://bofainstitute.cornell.edu/more/quantity-breeds-quality/. **Ideas found in *(Part 9, Process Over Perfection)***

2. Gross, Terry. "Comic Hari Kondabolu On 'The Simpsons' And The Problem With Apu." Fresh Air, NPR, 26 June 2018, https://www.npr.org/2018/06/26/623175387/comic-hari-kondabolu-on-the-simpsons-and-the-problem-with-apu .

3. Incite Coaching Academy. "Gibson-Banning Method." InciteCoachingAcademy.com, n.d., https://incitecoachingacademy.com. **General Concepts, Definitions and Distinctions found in *(Part 4, Values Over Strategies). Used with permission as a Certified Master Incite Coach.***

4. Kleon, Austin. *"Quantity leads to quality": The origin of a parable.* Austin Kleon's blog. Retrieved from. *December 10, 2020. https://austinkleon.com/2020/12/10/quantity-leads-to-quality-the-origin-of-a-parable/*

5. Martin, William. The Parent's Tao Te Ching: Ancient Advice for Modern Parents. Da Capo Press, 1997. **Quote found in *(Part 2 Become "Extra" at Being Ordinary)***

6. Reilly, Rick. "Gainesville State Football Gets the Best Gift of All." ESPN.com, 18 Dec. 2008, https://www.espn.com/espn/rickreilly/news/story?id=3789373. **Story found in *(Part 2 Become "Extra" at Being Ordinary)***

7. Tucker, Miriam. "Mirror, Mirror." Monitor on Psychology, vol. 36, no. 9, 2005, p. 64, https://www.apa.org/monitor/oct05/mirror#:~:text=They%20were%20first%20discovered%20in,primate%20grab%20the%20same%20object.

BOOKS & PODCASTS THAT INSPIRED THE MAGIC

BROWN, SUNNI. *THE DOODLE Revolution: Unlock the Power to Think Differently.* Portfolio/Penguin, 2014.

Clear, James. Atomic Habits: An Easy & Proven Way to Build Good Habits & Break Bad Ones. New York: Avery. 2018. **Ideas found in *Part 8 (Forced Achievement vs Inevitable Achievement), Part 9 (Weakness is a Gift That Allows Us to Create Processes)***

Crichton, Michael. *Jurassic Park.* Ballantine Books, 1990. p. 104. **Quote found in *Part 9 (Healing Our Ideas of Cycles and Time)***

Ford, Debbie. *The Dark Side of the Light Chasers: Reclaiming Your Power, Creativity, Brilliance, and Dreams.* Riverhead Books, 1998. **Ideas found in *Part 6: (Shadow)***

Gilbert, Elizabeth. *Big Magic: Creative Living Beyond Fear.* Riverhead Books, 2015. **Ideas found in *Part 4 (Two Geniuses), Part 10 (Everyone is a Creative Genius)***

Gladwell, Malcolm. The Tipping Point: How Little Things Can Make a Big Difference. New York: Little, Brown and Company. 2000. ***Part 8 (Forced Achievement vs Inevitable Achievement)***

Kleon, Austin. *Steal Like an Artist: 10 Things Nobody Told You About Being Creative.* Workman Publishing, 2012. **Just the most awesome book ever. Inspiration for the style and formatting of this book came from Kleon's book style.**

Northrup, Kate. Do Less: A Revolutionary Approach to Time and Energy Management for Busy Moms. Hay House, 2019. **Ideas found in , *Part 3 (Magic Void), Part 5 (Do Less), Part 9 (Healing Our Ideas of Cycles and Time)***

Phillips, Lacy. Expanded. Acast, 2017-2023. Audio podcast. **Ideas found in *Part 3 (Magic Void)***

Pressfield, Steven. The War of Art: Break Through the Blocks and Win Your Inner Creative Battles. New York: Warner Books. 2002. **Idea found in *Part 8 (Forced Achievement vs Inevitable Achievement)***

Tracy, Brian. *Eat That Frog!: 21 Great Ways to Stop Procrastinating and Get More Done in Less Time.* San Francisco, CA: Berrett-Koehler Publishers. 2001. **Idea found in *Part 8 (Eat the Frog)***

Illustrations

Stick Figure drawings by @zdeneksasek on Canva Pro

Compiled into Conceptual Drawings by Tessa Aranda

All other Photos & illustrations from Canva Pro or Unsplash edited by Tessa Aranda

About The Author

Tessa Aranda is a busy mom, wife, surfer, sunday-school teacher and friend living in gorgeous sunny San Diego. She is the Master of finding the Magic in Motherhood. With her podcast, books, and community "Mediocre Moms Club" she is building a space for moms that believe that intentional imperfection daily creates powerful moms and fun, fierce, love-filled families. She likes getting deep fast with new friends, and she swings from building complex marketing funnels and integrations to taking month long sabbaticals playing in the dirt with her kids. She's done doing what she's 'supposed to do' in life and business and she's never been happier. She helps women create more joy and ease in their businesses and lives through helping them magnify the "extra" in their ordinary. She's a Master Spark! Catalyst Coach, a speaker, author, and most Funcomfortable of all, a mom of 5 crazy creative kids.

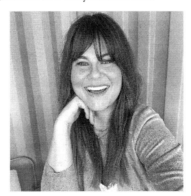

www.MediocreMomsClub.com

Made in the USA
Middletown, DE
10 March 2023

26529225R00077